Palliative Care

Editor

KIMBERLY A. CURSEEN

CLINICS IN
GERIATRIC MEDICINE

www.geriatric.theclinics.com

August 2023 • Volume 39 • Number 3

ELSEVIER

1600 John F. Kennedy Boulevard • Suite 1800 • Philadelphia, Pennsylvania, 19103-2899

http://www.theclinics.com

CLINICS IN GERIATRIC MEDICINE Volume 39, Number 3
August 2023 ISSN 0749–0690, ISBN-13: 978-0-443-13029-8

Editor: Taylor Hayes
Developmental Editor: Anita Chamoli

Clinics in Geriatric Medicine (ISSN 0749-0690) is published quarterly by Elsevier Inc., 360 Park Avenue South, New York, NY 10010-1710. Months of issue are February, May, August, and November. Business and Editorial Offices: 1600 John F. Kennedy Blvd., Suite 1800, Philadelphia, PA 191023-2899. Periodicals postage paid at New York, NY, and additional mailing offices. Subscription prices are $312.00 per year (US individuals), $748.00 per year (US institutions), $100.00 per year (US & Canadian student/resident), $340.00 per year (Canadian individuals), $946.00 per year (Canadian institutions), $444.00 per year (international individuals), $946.00 per year (international institutions), and $195.00 per year (international student/resident). Foreign air speed delivery is included in all *Clinics* subscription prices. All prices are subject to change without notice. POSTMASTER: Send address changes to *Clinics in Geriatric Medicine,* Elsevier Health Sciences Division, Subscription Customer Service, 3251 Riverport Lane, Maryland Heights, MO 63043. **Telephone: 1-800-654-2452 (U.S. and Canada); 314-447-8871 (outside U.S. and Canada). Fax: 314-447-8029. E-mail:** journalscustomerservice-usa@elsevier.com **(for print support) or** journalsonlinesupport-usa@elsevier.com **(for online support).**

Reprints. For copies of 100 or more, of articles in this publication, please contact the Commercial Reprints Department, Elsevier Inc., 360 Park Avenue South, New York, New York 10010-1710. Tel.: 212-633-3874; Fax: 212-633-3820, E-mail: reprints@elsevier.com.

Clinics in Geriatric Medicine is covered in *MEDLINE/PubMed (Index Medicus), EMBASE/Excerpta Medica, Current Contents/Clinical Medicine (CC/CM),* and the *Cumulative Index to Nursing & Allied Health Literature.*

Contributors

EDITOR

KIMBERLY A. CURSEEN, MD, FAAHPM
Director of Outpatient Supportive Care, Emory Palliative Care Center; Director of Winship Palliative Medicine Program, Associate Professor, Division of Palliative Medicine, Atlanta, Georgia

AUTHORS

REV. MATTHEW BAUHOF, MDiv
Oncology Chaplain, Division of Solid Tumor Oncology, Supportive and Palliative Oncology, University Hospitals Seidman Cancer Center, Cleveland, Ohio

YVAN BEAUSSANT, MD, MSc
Instructor in Medicine, Harvard Medical School, Department of Psychosocial Oncology and Palliative Care, Dana-Farber Cancer Institute, Atlanta, Georgia

SIVAN BEN-MOSHE, MD
Department of Medicine, Division of General Medicine and Geriatrics, Assistant Professor, Emory University School of Medicine, Senior Physician, Geriatrics Clinic, Emory Healthcare, Course Director of Geriatrics and Palliative Medicine M1 Emory SOM, Atlanta, Georgia

COLLEEN CARROLL, APRN-CNP
Certified Nurse Practitioner, Division of Solid Tumor Oncology, Supportive and Palliative Oncology, University Hospitals Seidman Cancer Center, Cleveland, Ohio

LAUREN CHIEC, MD
Assistant Professor of Medicine, Division of Solid Tumor Oncology, Case Western Reserve University School of Medicine, University Hospitals Seidman Cancer Center, Cleveland, Ohio

SARAH H. CROSS, PhD, MSW, MPH, MPH
Instructor, Division of Palliative Medicine, Department of Family and Preventive Medicine, Emory University, Atlanta, Georgia

KIMBERLY A. CURSEEN, MD, FAAHPM
Director of Outpatient Supportive Care, Emory Palliative Care Center; Director of Winship Palliative Medicine Program, Associate Professor, Division of Palliative Medicine, Atlanta, Georgia

MONA GUPTA, MD, AGSF, FAAHPM
Associate Professor of Medicine, Division of Solid Tumor Oncology, Case Western Reserve University School of Medicine, University Hospitals Seidman Cancer Center, Supportive and Palliative Oncology, Cleveland, Ohio

AUGUSTIN JOSEPH, MD
Instructor, Section of Palliative Medicine, Department of Medicine, Johns Hopkins Medical Institutions, Baltimore, Maryland

DIO KAVALIERATOS, PhD
Associate Professor and Director of Research and Quality, Division of Palliative Medicine, Department of Family and Preventive Medicine, Emory University, Atlanta, Georgia

LAWSON J. MARCEWICZ, MD
Department of Veterans Affairs, Atlanta Veterans Affairs Health Care System, Decatur, Georgia; Division of Palliative Medicine, Department of Family and Preventive Medicine, Emory University School of Medicine, Atlanta, Georgia

CHRISTINE MIKLOSOVIC, RN-BSN, CHPCA
Certified Nurse Partner, Division of Solid Tumor Oncology, Supportive and Palliative Oncology, University Hospitals Seidman Cancer Center, Cleveland, Ohio

KABIR NIGAM, MD, MRes
Resident Physician, Department of Psychiatry, Brigham and Women's Hospital, Harvard Medical School, Boston, Massachusetts

LYNN B. O'NEILL, MD
Department of Veterans Affairs, Atlanta Veterans Affairs Health Care System, Decatur, Georgia; Division of Palliative Medicine, Department of Family and Preventive Medicine, Emory University School of Medicine, Atlanta, Georgia

CYNTHIA OWUSU, MD, MS
Associate Professor of Medicine, Division of Solid Tumor Oncology, Case Western Reserve University School of Medicine, University Hospitals Seidman Cancer Center, Cleveland, Ohio

NAFIISAH B.M.H. RAJABALEE, MBBS
Fellow in Hospice and Palliative Medicine, Johns Hopkins School of Medicine, Baltimore, Maryland

LORI RUDER, DNP, APRN-CNP, AGACNP-BC, ACHPN
Certified Nurse Practitioner, Division of Solid Tumor Oncology, Supportive and Palliative Oncology, University Hospitals Seidman Cancer Center, Cleveland, Ohio

LAUREN E. SIGLER, MD
Department of Veterans Affairs, Atlanta Veterans Affairs Health Care System, Decatur, Georgia; Division of Palliative Medicine, Department of Family and Preventive Medicine, Emory University School of Medicine, Atlanta, Georgia

THOMAS J. SMITH, MD, FACP, FASCO, FAAHPM
Professor, Departments of Medicine and Oncology, Johns Hopkins Medical Institutions, Baltimore, Maryland

JABEEN TAJ, MD
Assistant Professor, Division of Hospice and Palliative Medicine, Department of Family Medicine, Emory University School of Medicine, Emory University Hospital, Atlanta, Georgia

COREY X. TAPPER, MD, MS
Assistant Professor, Department of Medicine, Johns Hopkins University School of Medicine, Assistant Professor, Section of Palliative Medicine, Department of Medicine, Johns Hopkins Medical Institutions, Baltimore, Maryland

EMILY PINTO TAYLOR, MD
Assistant Professor of Medicine, Division of Hospice and Palliative Medicine, Department of Family and Preventative Medicine, Division of General Internal Medicine, Department of Internal Medicine, Emory University School of Medicine, Grady Hospital, Atlanta, Georgia

CRISTINA VELOZZI-AVEROFF, MD
Clinical Fellow, Division of Hospice and Palliative Medicine, Department of Family and Preventative Medicine, Emory University School of Medicine, Atlanta, Georgia

BALAKRISHNA VEMULA, MD
Fellow, Departments of Medicine and Emergency Medicine, Johns Hopkins Medical Institutions, Baltimore, Maryland

THERESA VETTESE, MD
Associate Professor of Medicine, Division of General Internal Medicine, Department of Internal Medicine, Emory University School of Medicine, Atlanta, Georgia

Contents

> LGBTQ+ patients encounter discrimination and bias in health care settings. They experience worse health outcomes than their cisgender and heterosexual counterparts. There are numerous ways to provide equitable and comprehensive palliative care to seriously ill LGBTQ+ individuals. These strategies include communication techniques, encouragement to complete advance directives, implicit bias training, and interdisciplinary collaboration.

> Heart failure remains a condition with high morbidity and mortality affecting 23 million people globally with a cost burden equivalent to 5.4% of the total health care budget in the United States. These costs include repeated hospitalizations as the disease advances and care that may not align with individual wishes and values. The coincidence of comorbid conditions with advanced heart failure poses significant challenges in the geriatric population. Advance care planning, medication education, and minimizing polypharmacy are primary palliative opportunities leading to specialist palliative care such as symptom management at end of life and timing of referral to hospice.

> Palliative care is no longer synonymous with end-of-life care, and because supply has been well outstripped by demand, much of the practice of palliative care early in a patient's illness journey will take place in the primary care clinic—referred to as primary palliative care. Referral to specialty palliative care for complex symptom management or clarification on decision-making is appropriate, and can facilitate hospice referral, if indicated and in line with patient/family goals.

> Meeting the needs of people at the end of life (EOL) is a public health (PH) concern, yet a PH approach has not been widely applied to EOL care. The design of hospice in the United States, with its focus on cost containment, has resulted in disparities in EOL care use and quality. Individuals with

non-cancer diagnoses, minoritized individuals, individuals of lower socio-economic status, and those who do not yet qualify for hospice are particularly disadvantaged by the existing hospice policy. New models of palliative care (both hospice and non-hospice) are needed to equitably address the burden of suffering from a serious illness.

for optimum care. The importance of incorporating geriatric and palliative concerns in assessment, as well as early involvement of the multidiscipli-nary team, is discussed as a manner of addressing the needs of older adults with cancer. Concerns related to metabolic changes that can occur with aging, as well as risk for polypharmacy and inappropriate prescribing for older adults, are also reviewed.

In the older adult with a serious illness, the goal of palliative medicine and symptom management is to optimize quality of life. Frailty has become an overarching finding in many older adults with serious illness. Symptom management options need to be considered in the lens of increasing frailty along an illness trajectory. Here, the authors emphasize literature updates and best practices for the most common symptoms experienced by the older adult with a serious illness.

Global palliative medicine is a priority for global health. The aging world population lives with multiple chronic diseases and malignancies that often lead to debility, morbidity, mortality, and decreased quality of life. In the United States, 68% of adults aged older than 65 years live with 2 or more chronic conditions. Endeavors to improve access to palliative care for seniors are ongoing within "age-friendly health systems." This review article aims to provide an overview of the present state of global geriatric palliative care and to identify potential areas for future improvement.

Palliative Care

CLINICS IN GERIATRIC MEDICINE

ISSUES OF RELATED INTEREST

Medical Clinics of North America
https://www.medical.theclinics.com/
Primary Care: Clinics in Office Practice
https://www.primarycare.theclinics.com/
Critical Care Nursing Clinics
https://www.criticalcare.theclinics.com/

THE CLINICS ARE AVAILABLE ONLINE!
Access your subscription at:
www.theclinics.com

Preface

Advancing the Vision of Palliative Care for the Older Adult

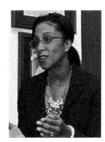

Kimberly A. Curseen, MD, FAAHPM
Editor

Aging is not a serious illness; it is a natural part of life. In this current era where ageism is openly promoted and practiced in our society, it is important to not conflate the process of natural aging with a disease. However, as treatments for serious illnesses have advanced and can provide longer lives, people, including our elders, may live with serious illnesses longer. Illness, like cancer, has become a disease of aging. It is important for primary care providers, geriatricians, and palliative care specialists to be prepared to meet the palliative care needs of these patients and families. There will not be enough palliative care or geriatric palliative care specialists to meet the demand. All providers who care for older adults, in any capacity, will need primary palliative care skills.

The demand for palliative care support is expected to grow, as it has for other populations. This special journal is devoted to exploring the intersection of geriatrics and palliative care, as well as the various challenges faced by practitioners in this area, as well as offering practical solutions to these challenges. Both palliative care and geriatrics have their foundations in the philosophy of shared decision making, the preservation and improvement of quality of life, and respect for patient values and choices.[1,2] Palliative and geriatric medicine can work together synergistically to address how older patients not only die with serious illnesses, but how they can live with an acceptable quality of life while living with these illnesses. The palliative approach to chronic, serious illnesses, such as Parkinson, dementia, and heart failure, can improve function, reduce unnecessary hospitalization and placement, and address the issues of polypharmacy and deprescribing in a personalized, patient-centered way with a focus on quality of life and symptom mitigation.[1,3] This approach has been proven to improve quality of life, decrease hospitalization and length of stay, and reduce financial toxicity.

Clin Geriatr Med 39 (2023) xi–xii
https://doi.org/10.1016/j.cger.2023.06.002
0749-0690/23/© 2023 Published by Elsevier Inc.

This journal offers a holistic view of how to recognize the palliative care needs of the elderly, as well as provides evidence-based approaches for providing care to this population. The diversity of geriatric palliative care is wide, and the chosen topics aim to introduce new subjects not commonly discussed in this field, while also offering updates on standard topics.

In addition to focusing on direct patient care, this journal addresses the policies and institutional barriers, as well as health inequities that impact palliative care delivery to older adults, both nationally and globally. Having this knowledge will enable providers to better understand and navigate the structural and institutional ageism that often hinders providing palliative care to this population, such as lack of social support, access to providers with expertise in symptom management, lack of access to symptom management medication, and provider and societal biases.[4,5] The intersectionality of older adults' ethnicity, race, gender, age, and socioeconomic status cannot be separated from the discussion of how palliative care is provided. This issue weaves addressing diversity, equity, and inclusion not just as separate topics, but as part of the topics that are covered.

We hope that this journal will help providers and clinicians better understand the complexities of geriatric palliative care through the selected topics and help them provide the highest quality of care to their patients. We are grateful for the authors who have contributed to this special journal and are excited to bring it to you. We look forward to the enriching conversations that it will bring.

Kimberly A. Curseen, MD, FAAHPM
Director of Outpatient Supportive Care
Emory Palliative Care Center
Director of Winship
Palliative Medicine Program Associate Professor
Division of Palliative Medicine
1821 Clifton Road, NE Suite 1017
Atlanta, GA 30329, USA

E-mail address:
kacurseen@emory.edu

REFERENCES

1. Voumard R, Rubli Truchard E, Benaroyo L, et al. Geriatric palliative care: a view of its concept, challenges and strategies. BMC Geriatr 2018;18:1–6.
2. Lazris A. Geriatric palliative care. Prim Care 2019;46(3):447–59.
3. Meira Erel E-LM, Dekeyser-Ganz F. Barriers to palliative care for advanced dementia: a scoping review. Ann Palliat Med 2017;6(4):365–79.
4. Aldridge MD, Hasselaar J, Garralda E, et al. Education, implementation, and policy barriers to greater integration of palliative care: a literature review. Palliat Med 2016;30(3):224–39.
5. Nelson KE, Wright R, Fisher M, et al. A call to action to address disparities in palliative care access: a conceptual framework for individualizing care needs. J Palliat Med 2021;24(2):177–80.

Geriatric Palliative Care
Providing Excellent Care to Lesbian, Gay, Bisexual, Transgender, Queer Older Adults

Corey X. Tapper, MD, MS

KEYWORDS

- LGBTQ+ • Sexual orientation and gender identity (SOGI)
- Sexual/gender minorities (SGM) • Geriatric palliative care • Health disparities

KEY POINTS

- The health needs of LGBTQ+ people are diverse and currently inadequately addressed.
- LGBTQ+ elders have little confidence that they will receive unbiased, competent, and inclusive care.
- Advance care planning, including the selection of a health care agent, is essential in the LGBTQ+ community given a historic reliance on chosen family which serves as a support and advocate.
- Equitable care for the LGBTQ+ community starts with cultural awareness and humility. Implicit bias training is critical for all health care workers.

INTRODUCTION

Along with other nations, the Unites States' population is aging.[1] By 2030, those aged 65 years and older will make up one-fifth of the US population. Although likely an underestimate, sexual and gender minorities (SGM) comprise 7.1% of our population as of 2021, which increased from 5.6% in 2020.[2] About one-quarter of SGMs in the United States are over 50 years old.[3] This statistic will continue to rise over the coming years as the Baby Boomer (those born during 1946–1964) and Gen X (those born during 1965–1980) generations age and is expected to double by the conclusion of this decade.[4,5] It is of utmost importance to ensure that LGBTQ+ individuals receive inclusive and competent medical care that is equitable to the general population, including palliative and end-of-life care for those with serious illnesses. Providers who care for older adults must have the knowledge, training, and skills to appropriately care for LGBTQ+ elders.

Department of Medicine, Johns Hopkins University School of Medicine, 1830 East Monument Street, Suite 8021, Baltimore, MD 21205, USA
E-mail address: ctapper1@jh.edu

Clin Geriatr Med 39 (2023) 359–368
https://doi.org/10.1016/j.cger.2023.04.001
0749-0690/23/© 2023 Elsevier Inc. All rights reserved.

NATURE OF THE PROBLEM

LGBTQ+ individuals face significant and unique health challenges compared to their cisgender and heterosexual counterparts. They also experience distinctive legal challenges and surrogacy issues. Their identity places them at varying degrees of social and cultural marginality.[6] Cultural marginality refers to the experience of living between two or more cultures without the ability to fully immerse oneself into any of them. A bias is an attitude toward a person/group of people or the association of stereotypes with them. Without conscious knowledge, bias is referred to as implicit. This is contrasted with explicit bias, in which a person is cognizant of their beliefs and actions. LGBTQ+ people are at high risk of experiencing both implicit and explicit bias in health care settings. This stems, in part, from a lack of cultural humility and awareness by health care providers. Cultural humility is a process of self-reflection which helps us to nurture relationships and through which we learn about our own cultures as well as the cultures and beliefs of those who have differing lived experiences.[7]

There is a relative lack of educational opportunities for medical professionals in this domain.[8,9] Medical providers, including trainees and independent practitioners, lack knowledge regarding the appropriate care of LGBTQ+ patients and the resources available to them. As such, there is an unfamiliarity among medical providers of the resources that are available to this population.[10] Further, data on sexual orientation and gender identity (SOGI) are not universally collected in clinical or research settings. This is especially true for LGBTQ+ elders, as most SGM research is conducted on younger individuals. These factors promote the continued invisibility of the LGBTQ+ community, including the LGBTQ+ geriatric community, whose needs may not be met in the traditional health care system.

When considering LGBTQ+ identity, there are three important topics to define.

- First, the LGBTQ+ population is heterogeneous and diverse, made up of varying SGM. This is also known as *minorities within a minority.* Individuals in this population have different health needs based on their gender identity and sexual orientation. Certainly, they can have markedly different lived experiences when compared to each other and their sexual- and gender-normative counterparts.
- Second is the concept of intersectionality, which is the convergence of internal and external factors that shape a person's lived experience.[11-13] These factors influence every aspect of their lives and lead to varying levels of bias against them. For example, an older LatinX transgender woman who identifies as a lesbian and has human immunodeficiency virus (HIV) may experience multiple forms of discrimination including ageism, racism, transphobia, sexism, homophobia, and nosophobia (fear of contracting a disease).
- Third is the model of a *chosen family.* Although social support for LGBTQ+ rights is steadily increasing, this is a relatively new phenomenon. The LGBTQ+ community cannot always rely on biological relatives for support. Further, they have fewer children, which leads to more limited caregiving resources with aging.[14] Therefore, they rely on other loved ones who may or may not be biologically related as their chosen family. This chosen family can provide support, love, caregiving, guidance, and community.

LGBTQ+ people have historically encountered many societal impediments to living as their true selves. Due to the marginalized status of many LGBTQ+ individuals, they are disproportionately affected by the provision and optimal access to appropriate medical care.[11] LGBTQ+ individuals have decreased access to insurance, food, transportation, and safe housing compared to their cisgender and heterosexual counterparts.[15,16] This is an effect of the structural discrimination that has been woven into our society, institutions, policies, and laws over the course of many years. This structural discrimination is also present in other marginalized populations.

Overt discrimination by medical providers leads to mistrust.[10] Explicit discrimination may arise in the form of inadequate, disrespectful, or abusive care.[10] One study showed that ~25% of palliative care team members witnessed overt discrimination of patients and/or caregivers.[17] Over half of the patients identifying as lesbian, gay, or bisexual were more likely to experience discrimination than their heterosexual and cisgender counterparts who were being cared for by the same palliative care team. Further, this was the case for over 60% of transgender individuals and the chosen family of LGBTQ+ individuals.[17]

Studies have shown that older LGBTQ+ people have little confidence that they will receive unbiased, competent, and inclusive care.[18] A recent review uncovered concerns that LGBTQ+ people have in health care settings.[19] As a whole, the LGBTQ population fears stigma, discrimination, and mistreatment in medicalized settings, which can be manifested actively, as previously discussed, or passively via lack of recognition and support. People of transgender experience frequently encounter insensitivity, especially regarding the acknowledgment of their gender. They also fear loss of independence due to disability or serious illness. When planning for death, transgender individuals must also make explicit directives to ensure that they are buried as the gender they identify with.

A study of focus groups in Canada revealed fear among LGBTQ+ elders of entering long-term care facilities, which may be necessary due to disability and/or serious illness.[18] The specific concerns revolve around isolation, loss of independence and decision-making capacity, and exposure to potentially unsafe environments—all falling under the umbrella of LGBTQ-related stigma. The possibility of loss of self-advocacy reveals a fear of not being able to live as one's true self and being "forced back into the closet". Previous data have shown that up to 75% of older LGBTQ+ people go back into the closet during such significant transitions due to concern for discrimination.[15] Lesbians fear isolation, poverty, and loss of solidarity among other women.[19] Potential social isolation and loneliness become more pertinent for LGBTQ+ elders as their circle of support dwindles with advancing age. This facet came into sharp focus during the height of the COVID-19 pandemic and also led to disenfranchised grief when members of someone's chosen family died.[6] This focus group also supports the need for more widespread advance care planning before loss of decision-making capacity.[18]

CLINICAL RELEVANCE

Due to mistrust of health care settings, SGM may delay care.[5,6] They also may be reluctant to disclose SOGI data due to concerns about bias. This is especially true for LGBTQ+ elders, 82% of whom have reported being verbally or physically victimized at some point in their lives.[20] There is a higher risk of substance use disorder among LGBTQ+ people compared to the general population.[21,22] Although all SGM have higher rates of depression, the prevalence is highest in transgender individuals.[23] Transgender women specifically have a higher incidence of mental health issues and immunodeficiency disorders.[24] Bisexual and lesbian older women are more likely to engage in high-risk health behaviors such as smoking and heavy alcohol use. This is also true of older bisexual and gay men. Older bisexual and gay men more frequently engage in risky sexual behavior.[20,25] Compared to cisgender and heterosexual women, LGBTQ+ women have an increased risk of coronary artery disease, obesity, and gynecologic and breast malignancies. Compared to cisgender and heterosexual men, LGBTQ+ men have an increased risk of cardiovascular disease, hypertension, diabetes, physical disability, and psychological distress.[20,26] Finally, older bisexual men and older transgender adults have poorer overall physical health compared to older gay men and older cisgender adults, respectively.[26]

PROTECTIVE FACTORS

Despite the bias and discrimination that SGM have historically experienced—and perhaps even because of this—the LGBTQ+ community has developed strategies to overcome adversity through resilience and self-reliance. Resilience involves the successful and positive management of internal and external stressors.[27] One example of resilience in the LGBTQ+ community is the interweaving of social networks that serve as support systems and bolster the value of all individuals in the community. Tangible examples include LGBTQ+ community centers and hotlines.[27]

LGBTQ+ individuals are also very mindful and careful in legal and financial matters.[5,14] In the literature, this is portrayed as robustness. LGBTQ+ elders also participate in behaviors that promote improved health including abstinence from substances, increased physical activity, and participation in spiritual and religious activities.[11,23] There is often a misconception that SGM do not participate in organized religious activities due to past and present discrimination leading to oppression and denial of rights such as marriage. However, there are several organized religions that have welcomed the LGBTQ+ community and have extended equitable rights to them. Qualitative research on LGBTQ+ elders has shown significant spirituality. This spirituality can take several forms, such as belief in a higher power, belief in community, and spirituality in oneself or one's chosen family.[28]

These positive behaviors can improve overall health, sense of well-being, regulate blood pressure, mitigate functional disability, and regulate body fat.[11,23] Further research on frailty in LGBTQ+ elders would be impactful as very limited data currently exist.

ADVANCE CARE PLANNING

Although advance care planning (ACP) is important for the general population, there are several reasons why it is essential for SGM. One survey showed robust familiarity with ACP among SGM, with 90% of respondents being familiar with living wills; 72% of respondents understood the importance of designating a health care agent. However, only 38% completed a living will, with 42% designating a medical decision-maker/proxy.[29] Another survey showed that 73% of LGBTQ+ people have discussed end-of-life preferences and just 42% had completed a formal advance directive.[14] Before state laws allowing for marriage equality and ultimately obtaining national recognition via the United States Supreme Court in the *Obergefell v Hodges* decision of 2015, SGM had unique challenges when advocating for themselves in health care settings.[30] These included difficulty obtaining medical insurance through a same-sex spouse or long-term domestic partner, limitations on hospital visitation, and health care agent designations not being honored.

Discussions on ACP should be encouraged with all LGBTQ+ elders and should include decisions regarding health care agent/surrogate decision-maker designation, end-of-life care, organ/body donation, funeral planning, and disposition of remains.[11,29] Please see **Table 1** for suggestions regarding communication strategies that can be used when discussing these topics.[31]

Table 1 Communication strategies when discussing advance care planning	
Communication Strategy	Examples
Normalize	"I speak to all of my patients about what is important to them and the type of care they would want in the future if they became sick."
Explore Values	"As you look to the future, what do you hope to accomplish?" "Were you to become very sick, what quality of life would be unacceptable for you?" "Tell me about what is most important to you."
Summarize Values	"You have given me a lot of useful information. What I am hearing is..."
Recommendation	"Based on your goals and values, I recommend... How does that sound?"

Developed by Corey X. Tapper, MD MS.

RECOMMENDATIONS

Our goal must be to ensure that LGBTQ+ individuals receive inclusive and competent medical care that is equitable to the general population, including palliative and end-of-life care for those with serious illnesses. Given providers' lack of comfort and knowledge in providing LGBTQ-inclusive care, education is an integral part of the solution. The Accreditation Council for Graduate Medical Education (ACGME) governs residency and fellowship programs in the United States. They have developed milestones composed of six core competencies: patient care, medical knowledge, professionalism, interpersonal and communication skills, practice-based learning and improvement, and systems-based practice.[32] Recently, there has been a call for incorporating specific LGBTQ-inclusive care competencies into the ACGME milestone framework.[33] This would help to ensure that post-graduate medical trainees are receiving education on this topic. The proposed competencies include understanding the appropriate use of SOGI, identifying specific medical concerns for LGBTQ+ people with serious illness, legal and ethical considerations, identifying LGBTQ+ caregiving needs, and creating safe spaces for education and support.[33] Creating formal curricula on LGBTQ+ inclusive care can also be an important tool in providing this education to medical learners. These curricula must also include a focus on caring for LGBTQ+ older adults.

As SGM are at high risk of bias in health care settings,[9] it is crucial to provide training in both implicit and explicit bias to all medical professionals. This should also include instruction on cultural humility and awareness, as knowledge of the various cultures within SGM will aid in guiding appropriate and effective medical care. For example, a recent curriculum used with medical students incorporated implicit bias training while students were learning to take sexual histories from patients who identified as LGBTQ+. Students found this education improved their comfort with taking sexual histories in a non-judgmental and culturally aware manner.[34] Similar training on other LGBTQ-inclusive care domains is necessary on an ongoing basis for medical professionals.

Clinical researchers must more uniformly collect SOGI data. Also, SOGI data should be collected routinely in clinical intake forms. A universal collection of SOGI data will allow medical professionals to more accurately hone screening, interventions, and treatments for LGBTQ+ patients. In addition, this collection of data will help to build rapport and trust with SGM as they will be seen as visible and important members of society.

Box 1
LGBTQ-inclusive care recommendations

Communication Skills:
- Avoid assumptions about gendered language. If you are unsure, ask the patient. This can include asking a patient if they have a "spouse" or "partner" as opposed to a "husband" or "wife".[38]
- Greet new patients without gender markers (eg, – Mr, Ms, Sir, Ma'am)
- Apologize if you accidently misgender someone, keeping it sincere and discrete[40]
- Call people by their preferred names and chart accordingly
- Use preferred pronouns
- Use body language and words that show non-judgment and acceptance
- Mirror patient language

Culturally Competent Care:
- Recognize the difference between sex assigned at birth and gender
- Avoid heteronormative language
- Explore sexual and intimacy needs[5]
- Address insurance barriers, especially when considering transgender health needs

Psychosocial Assessment:
- Questions about one's transition or genitals should only be asked when medically necessary
- Explore spiritual and/or religious beliefs and values
- Inquire about the family of choice and other support systems

Interdisciplinary:
- Speak up if you hear a colleague acting in a discriminatory way
- Intake forms should reflect patient diversity
- Post a non-discrimination policy in the waiting area
- Become familiar with common terms used by the LGBTQ+ community
- Provide ongoing educational opportunities for staff
- Advocate for inclusion of SOGI data in the electronic medical record

---

As social isolation can have negative impacts on mental health, routine screening for this is essential. The Patient Health Questionnaire-2 (PHQ-2) is an effective tool for screening for depression in all adult patients, including those who identify as LGBTQ+.[35] Loneliness, which is common among older patients, can be amplified in LGBTQ+ elders. This can be screened for using the University of California, Los Angeles (UCLA) Loneliness Scale[36] or the Three-Item Loneliness Scale.[37]

The language we use with LGBTQ+ patients should be open-ended, inviting, and non-judgmental. This will help to improve patient rapport, trust, and satisfaction. This will also help to promote goal-concordant care. Patients' chosen families should be integrated into care as much as patients wish, especially when it pertains to ACP and health care agent designation. Finally, it is important to ask for permission when examining patients. This is especially crucial with transgender patients, as they can tell clinicians what areas to avoid or be sensitive of.[11] See **Box 1** for other pearls regarding LGBTQ-inclusive care[33,38–40] and see **Table 2** for educational resources.

SUMMARY

LGBTQ+ patients experience discrimination and bias in health care settings. Although this can be partially explained by various prejudices, it is also caused by a lack of provider knowledge on how to optimally care for these patients, as well as a lack of cultural sensitivity and humility. Subsequently, LGBTQ+ patients experience worse outcomes in their physical and mental health, which are also influenced by economic hardship, underinsurance, relative paucity of advocacy, and delay in care due to mistrust of health care settings. There are concrete strategies that can be

Table 2
LGBTQ-inclusive care educational resources

https://implicit.harvard.edu	Harvard Implicit Association Test
https://prevention.ucsf.edu/transhealth/resources	UCSF Center of Excellence for Transgender Health
https://wpath.org/	World Professional Association for Transgender Health
https://cancer-network.org/	National LGBT Cancer Network
https://www.lambdalegal.org/sites/default/files/final_pp_ttp-2014-07_protecting-your-wishes-for-your-funeral.pdf	Lambda Legal Tools for Life and Financial Planning
https://www.mountsinai.org/files/MSHealth/Assets/HS/Locations/2021-Terminology-for-Sinai-Cheat-Sheet.pdf	Mount Sinai Center for Transgender Medicine and Surgery
https://fenwayhealth.org/the-fenway-institute/lgbtqia-aging-project/	LGBTQIA+ Aging Project
https://www.lgbtqiahealtheducation.org/	National LGBTQIA+ Health Education Center
LGBTQ-Inclusive Hospice and Palliative Care: A Practical Guide to Transforming Your Practice	Kimberly Acquaviva, PhD, MSW, CSE

implemented to provide equitable and comprehensive palliative care to seriously ill LGBTQ+ individuals. These strategies include communication techniques, encouragement to complete advance directives, implicit bias training, and interdisciplinary collaboration. In the future, more research should be focused on the health needs and outcomes of SGM, especially LGBTQ+ elders.

CLINICS CARE POINTS

- LGBTQ+ individuals represent at least 7.1% of the Unites States' population. This percentage has been steadily increasing over the last several decades. About a quarter of these are over 50 year old. As the Baby Boomer generation ages, the proportion of LGBTQ+ elders will increase significantly.
- SGM are at high risk of implicit and explicit bias in health care settings due to a lack of medical professionals' cultural awareness and relevant medical knowledge.
- LGBTQ+ people have historically had worse physical and mental health outcomes due to multiple factors including inadequate health care, underinsurance, delay in care, and economic hardship.
- There are many resources for education regarding LGBTQ-inclusive medical care, including palliative and end-of-life care. There are recent efforts to formalize LGBTQ-inclusive care competencies in graduate medical education.

DISCLOSURE

The author has nothing to disclose.

REFERENCES

1. Vespa J. The U.S. Joins Other Countries With Large Aging Populations. United States Census Bureau. Published March 13, 2018. Available at: https://www.

census.gov/library/stories/2018/03/graying-america.html. Accessed January 22, 2023.

2. Jones J. LGBT Identification in U.S. Ticks Up to 7.1%. The Gallup Organization. Published February 17, 2022. Available at: https://news.gallup.com/poll/389792/lgbt-identification-ticks-up.aspx. Accessed January 22, 2023.

3. LGBT Data & Demographics – The Williams Institute, UCLA Law School. LGBT Demographic Data Interactive. Published January 2019. Available at: https://williamsinstitute.law.ucla.edu/visualization/lgbt-stats/?topic=LGBT#demographic. Accessed January 22, 2023.

4. Choi S.K. and Meyer I.H., LGBT aging: a review of research findings, needs, and policy implications, 2016, The Williams Institute, UCLA School of Law. Available at: https://williamsinstitute.law.ucla.edu/publications/lgbt-aging/.

5. Stevens EE, Abrahm JL. Adding silver to the rainbow: palliative and end-of-life care for the geriatric LGBTQ patient. J Palliat Med 2019;22(5):602–6.

6. Rosa WE, Shook A, Acquaviva KD. LGBTQ+ inclusive palliative care in the context of COVID-19: pragmatic Recommendations for clinicians. J Pain Symptom Manage 2020;60(2):e44–7.

7. Yeager KA, Bauer-Wu S. Cultural humility: essential foundation for clinical researchers. Appl Nurs Res 2013;26(4). https://doi.org/10.1016/j.apnr.2013.06.008.

8. Daley AE, MacDonnell JA. Gender, sexuality and the discursive representation of access and equity in health services literature: implications for LGBT communities. Int J Equity Health 2011;10:40.

9. Sabin JA, Riskind RG, Nosek BA. Health care providers' implicit and explicit attitudes toward lesbian women and gay men. Am J Public Health 2015;105(9): 1831–41.

10. Maingi S, Radix A, Candrian C, et al. Improving the hospice and palliative care experiences of LGBTQ patients and their caregivers. Prim Care 2021;48(2): 339–49.

11. Javier NM. Palliative care needs, concerns, and affirmative strategies for the LGBTQ population. Palliat Care Soc Pract 2021;15. 26323524211039230.

12. Farmer DF, Yancu CN. Hospice and palliative care for older lesbian, gay, bisexual and transgender adults: the effect of history, discrimination, health disparities and legal issues on addressing service needs. Palliat Med Hosp Care Open J 2015; 1(2):36–43.

13. Quinn GP, Schabath MB, Sanchez J, et al. The importance of disclosure: lesbian, gay, bisexual, transgender/transsexual, queer/questioning, intersex (LGBTQI) individuals and the cancer continuum. Cancer 2015;121(8):1160–3.

14. Metlife mature market Institute®2, the lesbian and gay aging issues network of the American society on aging. Out and aging: the MetLife study of lesbian and gay Baby boomers. J GLBT Fam Stud 2010;6(1):40–57.

15. Espinoza R. Out & Visible: The Experiences and Attitudes of Lesbian, Gay, Bisexual and Transgender Older Adults, Ages 45-75. Services and Advocacy for GLBT Elder; 2014. Available at: https://www.sageusa.org/resource-posts/out-visible-the-experiences-and-attitudes-of-lesbian-gay-bisexual-and-transgender-older-adults-ages-45-75-by-the-numbers-full-report/. Accessed January 22, 2023.

16. Emlet CA. Social, economic, and health disparities among LGBT older adults. Generations 2016;40(2):16–22.

17. Stein GL, Berkman C, O'Mahony S, et al. Experiences of lesbian, gay, bisexual, and transgender patients and families in hospice and palliative care: perspectives of the palliative care team. J Palliat Med 2020;23(6):817–24.

18. Kortes-Miller K, Boulé J, Wilson K, et al. Dying in long-term care: perspectives from sexual and gender minority older adults about their fears and hopes for end of life. J Soc Work End-of-Life Palliat Care 2018;14(2–3):209–24.

19. Valenti KG, Jen S, Parajuli J, et al. Experiences of palliative and end-of-life care among older LGBTQ women: a review of current literature. J Palliat Med 2020; 23(11):1532–9.

20. Fredriksen-Goldsen KI, Kim HJ, Barkan SE, et al. Health disparities among lesbian, gay, and bisexual older adults: results from a population-based study. Am J Public Health 2013;103(10):1802–9.

21. Krehely J. How to Close the LGBT Health Disparities Gap. Center for American Progress; 2009. Available at: https://www.americanprogress.org/article/how-to-close-the-lgbt-health-disparities-gap/. Accessed January 22, 2023.

22. Cochran SD, Mays VM. Physical health complaints among lesbians, gay men, and bisexual and homosexually experienced heterosexual individuals: results from the California quality of life survey. Am J Public Health 2007;97(11):2048–55.

23. Fredriksen-Goldsen KI, Kim HJ, Shiu C, et al. Successful aging among LGBT older adults: physical and mental health-related quality of life by age group. Gerontol 2015;55(1):154–68.

24. Kenagy GP. Transgender health: findings from two needs assessment studies in philadelphia. Health Soc Work 2005;30(1):19–26.

25. Fredriksen-Goldsen KI, Kim HJ. The science of conducting research with LGBT older adults- an introduction to aging with pride: national health, aging, and sexuality/gender study (NHAS). Gerontol 2017;57(Suppl 1):S1–14.

26. Wallace SP, Cochran SD, Durazo EM, et al. The health of aging lesbian, gay and bisexual adults in California. Policy Brief UCLA Cent Health Policy Res 2011;(PB2011–2):1–8.

27. Meyer IH. Resilience in the study of minority stress and health of sexual and gender minorities. Psychology of Sexual Orientation and Gender Diversity 2015;2(3):209–13.

28. Fair TM. Lessons on older LGBTQ individuals' sexuality and spirituality for hospice and palliative care. Am J Hosp Palliat Care 2021;38(6):590–5.

29. Stein GL, Bonuck KA. Attitudes on end-of-life care and advance care planning in the lesbian and gay community. J Palliat Med 2001;4(2):173–90.

30. Kennedy A. Obergefell v. Hodges. Supreme Court of the United States; 2015:103. Available at: https://www.supremecourt.gov/DocketPDF/21/21-476/227884/20220614132338901_42501%20pdf%20Goldstein.pdf. Accessed January 15, 2023.

31. Tapper CX, Smith TJ. COVID-19 has put advance care planning in the spotlight. Here's how to talk to your patients. ASCO Daily News. Available at: https://dailynews.ascopubs.org/do/covid-19-has-put-advance-care-planning-spotlight-here-s-talk-your-patients. Accessed February 19, 2023.

32. Accreditation Council for Graduate Medical Education: Milestones. Available at: https://www.acgme.org/what-we-do/accreditation/milestones/overview/. Accessed January 24, 2023.

33. Liantonio J, Tapper CX, Danielewicz M, et al. A call for the creation of LGBTQ+ competencies for hospice and palliative medicine (HPM) fellowship programs. J Pain Symptom Manag 2022. https://doi.org/10.1016/j.jpainsymman.2022.12.009.

34. Mayfield JJ, Ball EM, Tillery KA, et al. Beyond men, women, or both: a comprehensive, LGBTQ-inclusive, implicit-bias-aware, standardized-patient-based

sexual history taking curriculum. MedEdPORTAL 2017;13:10634. https://doi.org/10.15766/mep_2374-8265.10634.

35. Kroenke K, Spitzer RL, Williams JBW. The patient health questionnaire-2: validity of a two-item depression screener. Medical Care 2003;41(11):1284.

36. Russell D, Peplau LA, Cutrona CE. The revised UCLA Loneliness Scale: concurrent and discriminant validity evidence. J Pers Soc Psychol 1980;39(3):472–80.

37. Hughes ME, Waite LJ, Hawkley LC, et al. A short Scale for measuring loneliness in large surveys: results from two population-based studies. Res Aging 2004; 26(6):655–72.

38. Dhawan N, Ovalle AA, Yeh JC. The role of hospice and palliative care in supporting and fostering trust among the LGBTQ+ population. Palliat Care Soc Pract 2021;15. 26323524211042636.

39. Barrett N, Wholihan D. Providing palliative care to LGBTQ patients. Nurs Clin 2016;51(3):501–11.

40. Acquaviva KD. LGBTQ-inclusive hospice and palliative care: a practical guide to transforming your practice. New York City, NY: Harrington Park Press; 2017.

End-Stage/Advanced Heart Failure

Geriatric Palliative Care Considerations

Jabeen Taj, MD[a],*, Emily Pinto Taylor, MD[b,c]

KEYWORDS

- Advanced/end stage heart failure • Elderly • Geriatric • Polypharmacy
- Comorbidities • Advance care planning • Primary palliative care
- Specialist palliative care

KEY POINTS

- Management of advanced heart failure in the geriatric population is challenging due to co-morbidities, limitations to advanced cardiac therapies, device management, and recurrent hospitalizations at end of life.
- Evidence based recommendations include integration of palliative care in the management of advanced heart failure along with traditional therapies to complement and facilitate treatment planning, mapping goals and advance care planning.
- End of life considerations include management of refractory symptoms and referral to hospice care to maintain dignity and relieve suffering.

INTRODUCTION AND SCOPE OF THE PROBLEM

Heart failure remains a condition with high morbidity and mortality affecting 23 million people globally with a cost burden equivalent to 5.4% of the total health care budget in the United States, roughly upward of $40 million annually. These costs include repeated hospitalizations as the disease advances, with 83% of Americans hospitalized at least once in their lifetime and 43% hospitalized 4 times.[1] The risk of hospitalization increases with risk factors such as age, poorly controlled hypertension, and

a Division of Hospice and Palliative Medicine, Department of Family Medicine, Emory University School of Medicine, Emory University Hospital, 1364 Clifton Road, Atlanta, GA 30322, USA; b Division of General Internal Medicine, Department of Family Medicine, Emory University School of Medicine, Grady Memorial Hospital, 80 Jesse Hill Drive Southeast, Atlanta, GA 30303, USA; c Division of Hospice and Palliative Medicine, Department of Family Medicine, Emory University School of Medicine, Grady Memorial Hospital, 80 Jesse Hill Drive Southeast, Atlanta, GA 30303, USA
* Corresponding author. Suite E244,1364 Clifton Road, Atlanta, GA 30322.
E-mail address: Jabeen.taj@emory.edu

Clin Geriatr Med 39 (2023) 369–378
https://doi.org/10.1016/j.cger.2023.04.010
0749-0690/23/© 2023 Elsevier Inc. All rights reserved.
geriatric.theclinics.com

Table 1
Challenges in management of advanced heart failure in older adults

Patient Factors	Provider Factors
Do not view as a life-limiting illness; the focus is on curative treatment	Do not view as a life-limiting illness; the focus is on guideline-directed therapy and preventing rehospitalizations
Lifestyle adjustment, polypharmacy, dietary restrictions	Advance care planning and discussing treatment preferences are delayed due to uncertainties in prognosis[8]
Poor quality of life, compliance issues, complex comorbidity[4]	Timing of palliative care consultation, when to refer to hospice[9,10]

comorbidities such as dementia, chronic kidney disease, diabetes, and chronic obstructive pulmonary disease.[2–4]

The coincidence of comorbid conditions with advanced/end-stage heart failure poses significant challenges in the geriatric population.[2,5,6] The pathophysiology of acute comorbidities such as infection and ischemia further affect the hemodynamics in this cohort of patients with limited cardiac reserve, resulting in acute decompensated heart failure.[2,5] Heart failure remains the leading cause of hospitalization in the elderly with 80% of Medicare beneficiaries (age 65 years and older) hospitalized in the last 6 months of life.[7]

Table 1 outlines the various patient and provider factors that can result in redundancy and care fragmentation.[8–10]

Examples of redundancy include polypharmacy, delay in referral to hospice after recurrent hospitalizations for advanced heart failure and/or multimorbidity, and uncertainty in prognostication.[5]

Although outcomes have improved with innovative medical and surgical management of advanced heart failure, mortality and rates of hospitalization/rehospitalization remain high, with almost 25% of older adults rehospitalized in 1 month and up to 70% rehospitalized in 1 year.[5,11] Although heart failure makes older adults vulnerable to rehospitalization, cause for rehospitalization is often comorbid illness unrelated to heart failure such as falls and infection.[11] Most older adults do not qualify for advanced heart failure therapies such as left ventricular assist device (LVAD) implantation and cardiac transplant due to stringent selection criteria—age, comorbidities, psychosocial barriers, and poor outcomes in aging adults. Compared with 84.5% of patients aged 55 years or younger who were discharged home, only 46.8% of adults aged 75 years or older survived a home discharge following LVAD implantation.[12]

Sex differences in end-of-life preferences were noted in the elderly heart failure population where women (mean age 83.4 years) were hospitalized less often than men (mean age 80.2 years) and received invasive interventions less commonly as well.[13] At least one study indicated that palliative care consultation reduces care transitions in heart failure by reducing the number of rehospitalization events and active in-hospital interventions such as mechanical ventilation and defibrillator implantation, all of which have significant implications in the aging heart failure patient.[14]

CONSIDERATIONS FOR PALLIATIVE CARE

Many challenges exist in the management of geriatric heart failure patients who may simultaneously suffer from frailty, cognitive decline, structural heart disease, and vascular conditions such as stroke and coronary artery disease.[1,5] Frailty, anorexia, cachexia, and sarcopenia are particularly prevalent in heart failure and are the harbingers of poor clinical outcomes ranging from increased health care utilization in the form of emergency department visits and hospitalizations at end of life to the more egregious such as falls, disability, cognitive decline, and higher mortality rates.[15] The pathophysiologic pathways linking heart failure and cognitive impairment include cerebral hypoperfusion, systemic inflammation, and neurohormonal dysregulation.[16] The Rush Memory Project (1588 dementia-free participants) demonstrated that a high cardiovascular risk burden may predict a decline in episodic memory, working memory, and perceptual speed with structural changes on brain imaging.[16,17] Channeling innovative treatments such as empagliflozin in the management of heart failure and diabetes can have beneficial effects on cognitive impairment by slowing estimated glomerular filtration rate decline and thereby positively affecting neurohormonal dysregulation.[18,19] The complexity and uncertain trajectory of illness can take a toll on the quality of life and detract from important shared decision-making and advance care planning conversations among patients, families, and specialty care teams.[4,8,14,20]

The incidence of sudden cardiac death remains substantial (300,000 to 400,000 deaths annually in the United States), and patients with progressive disease often need counseling about the life-limiting nature of this illness. Ventricular arrhythmias are common in severe heart failure accounting for a prevalence of 85% of cases.[21] The risk of these fatal arrhythmias can be significantly decreased with implantable cardioverter-defibrillators (ICDs) in populations most at risk—advanced heart failure patients with ischemic and/or dilated cardiomyopathy.[21] Risk stratification and shared decision-making on the benefits versus burdens of such treatments highlight the importance of goals of care discussions in the geriatric population.[22,23]

Palliative care can play a key role in reducing suffering through proactive goals-of-care conversations as well as atypical symptom management in older adults[9,10] (**Figs. 1 and 2, Table 2**).[4,6,20]

Polypharmacy is a well-known entity in the geriatric population, especially in the setting of recurrent admissions and discharges; this is evident in heart failure where not uncommonly, the incidence of polypharmacy increases with recurrent hospitalizations and worsening symptoms.[24,25] Elderly patients who were previously on less than 5 medications end up on more than 10 medications, not all of which are related to heart failure.[25]

Goals of care:
How do you like to receive information? Simple, straightforward, avoid negative information

What is most important to you?

Exploring hopes and worries

What are you willing to go through to achieve those goals? Tradeoffs

What makes life worth living for you? Exploring joy

Can you imagine a quality of life that would be unacceptable to you?

Have you thought about your goals if you got sicker?

Fig. 1. Goals of care in older adults with advanced heart failure.[56,57]

- Management of advanced heart failure in the geriatric population is challenging due to co-morbidities, limitations to advanced cardiac therapies, device management, and recurrent hospitalizations at end of life.
- Multiple studies recommend the integration of palliative care in the management of advanced heart failure along with traditional management to complement and facilitate treatment planning, mapping goals and advance care planning.
- Palliative care can particularly assist with nuanced goals of care discussions with disease progression, empathic support for the patient and caregiver, and atypical symptom management focusing on quality of life.
- End-of-life considerations include management of refractory symptoms and referral to hospice care to maintain dignity and relieve suffering.

Fig. 2. Clinical pearls.

Advance care planning, medication education, minimizing polypharmacy, and deprescribing are palliative opportunities, and multiple studies indicate the underutilization of palliative care in this group of patients.[3,12,26–28] **Table 3** summarizes the integration of palliative care in traditional heart failure management and impresses on the transition of a primary palliative approach (goals of care, advance care planning) to specialized supportive care (timing of hospice referral).[29]

DEVICE MANAGEMENT IN END-STAGE/ADVANCED HEART FAILURE

As patients with advanced congestive heart failure transition to the end of life, it is important for primary care physicians (PCPs) to consider the presence or absence of advanced cardiac therapies that may be used by the patient, including pacemakers, ICDs, external defibrillators ("life vests"), or LVADs.[30]

Management of LVADs, a form of circulatory support for the heart, is typically deferred to cardiologists with specialization in advanced heart failure, and it is unlikely that their deactivation would occur within the purview of the geriatric or primary care clinic. However, management of pacemakers, ICDs, and external defibrillators may be within the scope of a geriatric or primary care practice and therefore merits a broader discussion here.[31,32]

Epidemiology and Use

According to the American Heart Association, ICD insertions more than doubled in the United States, from 46,000 in 2001 to approximately 150,000 in 2011.[33] Pacemaker

Table 2 Symptom delineation in advanced heart failure[4,6,20]	
Typical Symptoms	**Atypical Symptoms**
Fatigue	Anorexia, cachexia, nausea, thirst
Dyspnea	Pain
Edema	Anxiety, depression
	Insomnia
	Delirium[a]
	Dyspnea refractory to diuretics[a]

[a] Terminal symptoms in end-stage heart failure.

Table 3
Transitions of care: integrating palliative care upstream and evolving to nuanced goals-of-care discussions including referral to hospice[29,36,37]

Traditional Heart Failure Management	Upstream Integration of Palliative Care
Guideline-directed medical therapy	Develop best practices to consult palliative care as early as the first presentation in adults aged 65 years and older
Consideration for advanced heart failure therapies (AHFT)	Longitudinal support: patients seen by palliative care consult service inpatient can benefit from outpatient follow-up
Palliative care is consulted if the patient is not a candidate for AHFT or repeated hospitalizations	Atypical symptom management, social and spiritual support—assess and address psychosocial and spiritual distress
Palliative care consultation can occur in conjunction with expert heart failure management—patient and provider education	Mapping and remapping of goals with each hospitalization as well as worsening disease trajectory
	Quality of life for patient and caregiver—therapy, respite options for caregiver fatigue and burnout including home palliative services
	Specialist care: referral to hospice

insertions increased from 177,000 to more than 200,000.[32] During this time, approximately 50% of ICDs and 85% of pacemakers were implanted in people older than 65 years.[30,32] Given the aging US population, it is expected that this number will continue to grow.

Patients with chronic heart failure with reduced ejection fraction are at an increased risk of sudden cardiac death due to ventricular arrhythmias.[31] ICDs are highly effective for the prevention of sudden cardiac death in selected patients known to be at high risk for life-threatening ventricular arrhythmias.[34,35] As a result, ICDs are indicated to be placed in these patients according to ESC guidelines when in line with goals, as well as predicted survival of more than 1 year with good functional status.[36] At times, patients will wear temporary external defibrillators ("life vests") for some time before the implantation of permanent, internal ICDs.[37,38] Both devices serve the same function—to monitor heart rhythm and terminate spontaneous and induced ventricular arrhythmias by automatic defibrillation shock delivery and, ideally, prolong life.[37]

Pacemakers were similarly designed to prolong life by treating abnormal tachyarrhythmias and bradyarrhythmias (cardiac resynchronization therapy); placement is indicated for patients who suffer from or are at risk of these conditions.[39,40]

Ethical Considerations in the Management of Advanced Cardiac Therapies at End of Life

Few review articles have included guidelines for palliative care specialists about management of these advanced therapies in the context of deactivation at the end of life. There is a gap in the literature for PCPs and geriatricians who manage these patients chronically and may engage in these conversations before referral to specialty palliative care occurs.[41–43] Management of these devices at the end of life involves both ethical and clinical considerations.

Ethically, although there has been consensus that deactivation of ICDs is a morally permissible act near the end of life, there has been some debate regarding the deactivation of pacemakers in terminally ill patients, with concern that deactivation of pacemaker function at the end of life could be interpreted as assisted dying.[44–50] In general, a patient's decision to decline or withdraw life-prolonging therapy at any time is consistent with the principle of respect for autonomy, which extends to both devices and reflects prevailing medical ethics.[51] Most medical ethicists do not consider a pacemaker as a part of a patient's self, and believe it can be withdrawn, similar to hemodialysis or mechanical ventilation.[52] Importantly, in the United States currently, there is no ethical or legal distinction between refusing cardiac device implantation (ICD or pacemaker) or requesting withdrawal of that device, provided this is desired by the patient.[45,46]

Clinical Considerations in Management of Advanced Cardiac Therapies at End of Life

In approaching end-of-life conversations in the realm of advanced heart failure and technology use, there are multiple considerations.

First, as discussed in more broad reviews of the role of geriatricians and PCPs in providing primary palliative care, these patients should engage in advance care planning and, ideally, complete advance directives that name a surrogate medical decision-maker. The authors encourage this to take place before any serious decompensation or medical emergency.[40,53,54]

Next, as recommended by the American College of Cardiology/American Heart Association (ACC), discussions of when to initiate, continue, and discontinue life-sustaining therapies such as ICDs and pacemakers should start at the time of implantation and long before functional capacity or outlook for survival is severely reduced.[43,50] Most tertiary care centers now include preparedness planning discussions before LVAD implantation to specifically address advance care planning and timing of device deactivation in circumstances of concomitant comorbidity (terminal metastatic cancer) or acute catastrophic complication (massive stroke)

Table 4	
Advance care planning considerations for cardiac devices in advanced heart failure	
Before placement	Consider informed consent before placement, with a focus on "when this device no longer helps me meet my goals."[48] Failure to do this can lead to increased suffering at the end of life.[49]
	Review the differences between pacemakers and ICDs with families and clarify that patients may still have a natural, painless death without pacemaker deactivation, should that be desired at the end of life.[59,60]
During times of severe illness/ decompensation	Review communication tools such as the Serious Illness Conversation Guide to discuss uncertainty and reconsideration of whether technology is helping to meet patient's goals, in the setting of changing medical realities and evolving goals of care.[56]
Before deactivation	Consider if referral to specialty palliative care may be indicated, palliative care consultation is helpful for patients interested in device deactivation and their primary care providers, without affecting survival.[60]

development.[55] Currently existing communication tools such as the Serious Illness Conversation Guide or Conversation Starter Guide may be helpful in facilitating these discussions and providing a framework for discussing prognosis, goals, and trade-offs.[56,57] ACC has developed apps such as CardioSmart and AMI Choice to improve patient education and empower patients to make informed choices.[22,23] Suggested topics pertinent to advanced heart failure and device management are listed in **Table 4**.[48,58–60]

It may be helpful for PCPs and geriatricians to review the process of discontinuation in order to guide these conversations, including utilization of a transcutaneous magnet to deactivate ICD function (while preserving pacemaker function if present) followed by electronic deactivation of the internal device.[50] Patients may have questions about the expected timeline before a fatal dysrhythmia, which differs by individual patient—prognostic conversations (in a patient without an active ICD) should involve the patient's cardiologist.

SUMMARY

Heart failure remains the leading cause of death due to its significant interplay with other life-limiting and chronic illnesses in older adults. Systematic collaboration between heart failure and palliative specialists can positively affect the trajectory of illness and guide informed decision-making in geriatric patients. The integration of palliative care in the plan of care can preserve dignity and reduce suffering in the patient with geriatric heart failure.[61,62]

DISCLOSURE

The authors have nothing to disclose.

REFERENCES

1. van Riet EE, Hoes AW, Wagenaar KP, et al. Epidemiology of heart failure: the prevalence of heart failure and ventricular dysfunction in older adults over time. A systematic review. Eur J Heart Fail 2016;18(3):242–52.
2. Forman DE, Ahmed A, Fleg JL. Heart failure in very old adults. Curr Heart Fail Rep 2013;10(4):387–400.
3. Butrous H, Hummel SL. Heart failure in older adults. Can J Cardiol 2016;32(9): 1140–7.
4. McClung JA. End-of-life care in the treatment of heart failure in older adults. Heart Failure Clin 2017;13(3):633–44.
5. Dharmarajan K, Dunlay SM. Multimorbidity in older adults with heart failure. Clin Geriatr Med 2016;32(2):277–89.
6. Gure TR, Blaum CS, Giordani B, et al. Prevalence of cognitive impairment in older adults with heart failure. J Am Geriatr Soc 2012;60(9):1724–9.
7. Panday A, Golwala H, Xu H, et al. Association of 30-day readmission metric for heart failure under the hospital readmissions reduction program with quality of care and outcomes. JACC Heart Fail 2016;4(12):935–46.
8. Lipinski M, Eagles D, Fischer LM, et al. Heart failure and palliative care in the emergency department. Emerg Med J 2018;35(12):726–9.
9. Okumura T, Sawamura A, Murohara T. Palliative and end-of-life care for heart failure patients in an aging society. Korean J Intern Med 2018;33(6):1039–49.
10. Romano M. [Palliative care and heart failure: is it time to talk?]. Recenti Prog Med 2018;109(4):216–9.

11. Dharmarajan K, Rich MW. Epidemiology, pathophysiology, and prognosis of heart failure in older adults. Heart Failure Clin 2017;13(3):417–26.

12. Caraballo C, DeFilippis EM, Nakagawa S, et al. Clinical outcomes after left ventricular assist device implantation in older adults: an INTERMACS analysis. JACC Heart Fail 2019;7(12):1069–78.

13. Van Spall HGC, Hill AD, Fu L, et al. Temporal trends and sex differences in intensity of healthcare at the end of life in adults with heart failure. J Am Heart Assoc 2021;10(1):e018495.

14. Diop MS, Bowen GS, Jiang L, et al. Palliative care consultation reduces heart failure transitions: a matched analysis. J Am Heart Assoc 2020;9(11):e013989.

15. Vitale C, Spoletini I, Rosano GM. Frailty in heart failure: implications for management. Card Fail Rev 2018;4(2):104–6.

16. Leto L, Feola M. Cognitive impairment in heart failure patients. J Geriatr Cardiol 2014;11(4):316–28.

17. Song R, Xu H, Dintica CS, et al. Associations between cardiovascular risk, structural brain changes, and cognitive decline. J Am Coll Cardiol 2020;75(20):2525–34.

18. Mone P, Lombardi A, Gambardella J, et al. Empagliflozin improves cognitive impairment in frail older adults with type 2 diabetes and heart failure with preserved ejection fraction. Diabetes Care 2022;45(5):1247–51.

19. Packer M, Butler J, Zannad F, et al. Effect of empagliflozin on worsening heart failure events in patients with heart failure and preserved ejection fraction: EMPEROR-preserved trial. Circulation 2021;144(16):1284–94.

20. Upadhya B, Kitzman DW. Heart failure with preserved ejection fraction in older adults. Heart Failure Clin 2017;13(3):485–502.

21. Lane RE, Cowie MR, Chow AW. Prediction and prevention of sudden cardiac death in heart failure. Heart 2005;91(5):674–80.

22. Krauskopf PB. Relief central with coronavirus guidelines and cardiosmart heart explorer apps. J Nurse Pract 2020;16(7):543–4.

23. Branda ME, Kunneman M, Meza-Contreras AI, et al. Shared decision-making for patients hospitalized with acute myocardial infarction: a randomized trial. Patient Prefer Adherence 2022;16:1395–404.

24. Skrzypek A, Mostowik M, Szeliga M, et al. Chronic heart failure in the elderly: still a current medical problem. Folia Med Cracov 2018;58(4):47–56.

25. Unlu O, Levitan EB, Reshetnyak E, et al. Polypharmacy in older adults hospitalized for heart failure. Circ Heart Fail 2020;13(11):e006977.

26. Bekelman DB, Hutt E, Masoudi FA, et al. Defining the role of palliative care in older adults with heart failure. Int J Cardiol 2008;125(2):183–90.

27. Diop MS, Rudolph JL, Zimmerman KM, et al. Palliative care interventions for patients with heart failure: a systematic review and meta-analysis. J Palliat Med 2017;20(1):84–92.

28. Widera E, Pantilat SZ. Hospitalization as an opportunity to integrate palliative care in heart failure management. Curr Opin Support Palliat Care 2009;3(4):247–51.

29. Kavalieratos D, Gelfman LP, Tycon LE, et al. Palliative care in heart failure: rationale, evidence, and future priorities. J Am Coll Cardiol 2017;70(15):1919–30.

30. Gregoratos G. Permanent pacemakers in older persons. J Am Geriatr Soc 1999;47(9):1125–35.

31. Breitenstein A, Steffel J. Devices in heart failure patients-who benefits from ICD and CRT? Front Cardiovasc Med 2019;6:111.

32. Greenspon AJ, Patel JD, Lau E, et al. Trends in permanent pacemaker implantation in the United States from 1993 to 2009: increasing complexity of patients and procedures. J Am Coll Cardiol 2012;60(16):1540–5.

33. Kremers MS, Hammill SC, Berul CI, et al. The National ICD Registry Report: version 2.1 including leads and pediatrics for years 2010 and 2011. Heart Rhythm 2013;10(4):e59–65.

34. Moss AJ, Hall WJ, Cannom DS, et al. Improved survival with an implanted defibrillator in patients with coronary disease at high risk for ventricular arrhythmia. Multicenter Automatic Defibrillator Implantation Trial Investigators. N Engl J Med 1996; 335(26):1933–40.

35. Moss AJ, Zareba W, Hall WJ, et al. Prophylactic implantation of a defibrillator in patients with myocardial infarction and reduced ejection fraction. N Engl J Med 2002;346(12):877–83.

36. Ponikowski P, Voors AA, Anker SD, et al. 2016 ESC Guidelines for the diagnosis and treatment of acute and chronic heart failure: the Task Force for the diagnosis and treatment of acute and chronic heart failure of the European Society of Cardiology (ESC). Developed with the special contribution of the Heart Failure Association (HFA) of the ESC. Eur J Heart Fail 2016;18(8):891–975.

37. Barraud J, Cautela J, Orabona M, et al. Wearable cardioverter defibrillator: bridge or alternative to implantation? World J Cardiol 2017;9(6):531–8.

38. Al-Khatib SM, Stevenson WG, Ackerman MJ, et al. 2017 AHA/ACC/HRS guideline for management of patients with ventricular arrhythmias and the prevention of sudden cardiac death: a report of the American college of Cardiology/American heart association task force on clinical practice guidelines and the heart rhythm society. J Am Coll Cardiol 2018;72(14):e91–220.

39. Epstein AE, DiMarco JP, Ellenbogen KA, et al. ACC/AHA/HRS 2008 guidelines for device-based therapy of cardiac rhythm abnormalities: a report of the American college of Cardiology/American heart association task force on practice guidelines (writing committee to revise the ACC/AHA/NASPE 2002 guideline update for implantation of cardiac pacemakers and antiarrhythmia devices) developed in collaboration with the American association for thoracic surgery and society of thoracic surgeons. J Am Coll Cardiol 2008;51(21):e1–62.

40. Lam PH, Taffet GE, Ahmed A, et al. Cardiac resynchronization therapy in older adults with heart failure. Heart Failure Clin 2017;13(3):581–7.

41. Morrison LJ, Calvin AO, Nora H, et al. Managing cardiac devices near the end of life: a survey of hospice and palliative care providers. Am J Hosp Palliat Care 2010;27(8):545–51.

42. Ezekowitz JA, Rowe BH, Dryden DM, et al. Systematic review: implantable cardioverter defibrillators for adults with left ventricular systolic dysfunction. Ann Intern Med 2007;147(4):251–62.

43. Heidenreich PA, Bozkurt B, Aguilar D, et al. 2022 AHA/ACC/HFSA Guideline for the management of heart failure: a report of the American College of Cardiology/American heart association joint committee on clinical practice guidelines. Circulation 2022;145(18):e895–1032.

44. Berger JT. The ethics of deactivating implanted cardioverter defibrillators. Ann Intern Med 2005;142(8):631–4.

45. England R, England T, Coggon J. The ethical and legal implications of deactivating an implantable cardioverter-defibrillator in a patient with terminal cancer. J Med Ethics 2007;33(9):538–40.

46. Quill TE, Barold SS, Sussman BL. Discontinuing an implantable cardioverter defibrillator as a life-sustaining treatment. Am J Cardiol 1994;74(2):205–7.

47. Wu EB. The ethics of implantable devices. J Med Ethics 2007;33(9):532–3.
48. Basta LL. End-of-life and other ethical issues related to pacemaker and defibrillator use in the elderly. Am J Geriatr Cardiol 2006;15(2):114–7.
49. Rhymes JA, McCullough LB, Luchi RJ, et al. Withdrawing very low-burden interventions in chronically ill patients. JAMA 2000;283(8):1061–3.
50. Benjamin MM, Sorkness CA. Practical and ethical considerations in the management of pacemaker and implantable cardiac defibrillator devices in terminally ill patients. SAVE Proc 2017;30(2):157–60.
51. Beauchamp IF, Childress TL. Nonmaleficence. In: Beauchamp TL, editor. Principles of biomedical ethics. Oxford (NY): Oxford University Press; 1994. p. 189–258.
52. Huddle TS, Amos Bailey F. Pacemaker deactivation: withdrawal of support or active ending of life? Theor Med Bioeth 2012;33(6):421–33.
53. Kolte D, Abbott JD, Aronow HD. Interventional therapies for heart failure in older adults. Heart Failure Clin 2017;13(3):535–70.
54. Brannstrom M, Fischer Gronlund C, Zingmark K, et al. Meeting in a 'free-zone': clinical ethical support in integrated heart-failure and palliative care. Eur J Cardiovasc Nurs 2019;18(7):577–83.
55. Swetz KM, Freeman MR, AbouEzzedine OF, et al. Palliative medicine consultation for preparedness planning in patients receiving left ventricular assist devices as destination therapy. Mayo Clin Proc 2011;86(6):493–500.
56. Labs, A. Serious Illness Conversation Guide. 2015. Available at: https://www.ariadnelabs.org/wp-content/uploads/2017/05/SI-CG-2017-04-21_FINAL.pdf. Accessed November 28, 2022.
57. Improvement, I.f.H. The Conversation Starter Guide. 2022. Available at: https://theconversationproject.org/wp-content/uploads/2020/12/ConversationStarterGuide.pdf. Accessed November 28, 2022.
58. Goldstein N, Carlson M, Livote E, et al. Brief communication: management of implantable cardioverter-defibrillators in hospice: a nationwide survey. Ann Intern Med 2010;152(5):296–9.
59. Hutchison K, Sparrow R. Ethics and the cardiac pacemaker: more than just end-of-life issues. EP Europace 2017;20(5):739–46.
60. Pasalic D, Gazelka HM, Topazian RJ, et al. Palliative care consultation and associated end-of-life care after pacemaker or implantable cardioverter-defibrillator deactivation. Am J Hosp Palliat Med 2016;33(10):966–71.
61. Hauptman PJ, Havranek EP. Integrating palliative care into heart failure care. Arch Intern Med 2005;165(4):374–8.
62. Bakitas M, Macmartin M, Trzepkowski K, et al. Palliative care consultations for heart failure patients: how many, when, and why? J Card Fail 2013;19(3):193–201.

Care Throughout the Journey–The Interaction Between Primary Care and Palliative Care

Emily Pinto Taylor, MD[a,b,*], Cristina Vellozzi-Averhoff, MD[a], Theresa Vettese, MD[b]

KEYWORDS

- Primary palliative care • Specialty palliative care • Advance care planning
- Opiate misuse

KEY POINTS

- Supply of palliative care physicians has been outstripped by demand, and some key symptom management will be based in a patient's primary care office.
- Primary palliative care assessment includes symptom assessment, assessment of patient distress, clarification on decision-makers, and advance care planning.
- Referral to specialty palliative care, when appropriate and available, improves quality of life and outcomes of care for patients.
- Primary care physicians must consider opiate use and misuse while continuing to prescribe opiate medications for cancer pain in the outpatient setting, including when to taper these medications.

INTRODUCTION

Scope and Definition of Palliative Care

Palliative care is often thought to be synonymous with end-of-life care but this is untrue. In fact, studies in the last 15 years have shown that the early involvement with palliative care may increase quality of life, decrease cost of care, and importantly, improve survival of patients with metastatic cancer despite less aggressive care at the end of life.[1,2]

Hospice and Palliative Medicine (HPM) was recognized as a subspecialty formally by the Accreditation Council for Graduate Medical Education (ACGME) in 2009, and

[a] Division of Hospice and Palliative Medicine, Department of Family and Preventative Medicine, Emory University School of Medicine, Atlanta, GA, USA; [b] Division of General Internal Medicine, Department of Internal Medicine, Emory University School of Medicine, Atlanta, GA, USA
* Corresponding author. Division of General Medicine, 49 Jesse Hill Jr. Drive. Atlanta, GA 30303.
E-mail address: epintotaylor@emory.edu

Clin Geriatr Med 39 (2023) 379–393
https://doi.org/10.1016/j.cger.2023.04.002
0749-0690/23/© 2023 Elsevier Inc. All rights reserved.

geriatric.theclinics.com

fellowship training is now required nationally for physicians interested in becoming board certified and practicing HPM. There has been steady growth in the number of HPM fellowships nationally during the past 5 years, with 156 programs currently in existence, representing 518 available slots for physician trainees in 2021.[3] Certifications now also exist for nurses, advanced practice providers, social workers, and chaplains working in palliative care.[4–6] Although initially palliative care was limited to the inpatient acute care setting, because of the increase in certified providers and the diversity of their practice patterns, palliative care programs have seen significant growth, and patients are often able to receive palliative care services in other settings—outpatient clinics, emergency departments, and different inpatient departments, to include critical care units.[7,8]

According to the Center to Advance Palliative Care, the focus of palliative care is to "provide patients with relief from the symptoms, pain, and stress of the serious illness, whatever the diagnosis, and improve the quality of life for patients and their families."[7] The American Society of Clinical Oncology expands this definition, noting more broadly that the goal of palliative care is "the relief of suffering, in all of its dimensions."[2] Our definition of palliative care is a blend of these—that palliative care focuses on managing symptoms (often difficult to control) while also facilitating communication between families and medical providers and discussion of appropriate goals of care, particularly for patients with advanced, life-limiting illness, or heavy symptom burden.

Why Primary Care Physicians Should Be Familiar with Palliative Care Approaches

In our aging population, the supply of palliative care physicians has already outstripped demand. Current estimates report 6600 board-certified physicians in practice, a projected shortage of 18,000 physicians (based on optimal need for specialists), and less than 250 fellowship-trained physicians entering the field annually.[9] It has been estimated that there will be no more than 1% absolute growth in palliative care physicians in 20 years, whereas during the same period, the number of people eligible for palliative care will grow by more than 20%—this is a ratio of only 1 physician for every 26,000 patients by 2030.[9] This highlights the importance of primary care physicians (PCPs) being trained as partners and extensions of the palliative care team. Partnership with PCPs to address basic aspects of palliative care in the primary care clinic is often referred to as "primary palliative care."

Primary palliative care involves basic communication and symptom management skills that are possessed by physicians of all specialties. It is distinguished from specialty palliative care (or "secondary palliative care"), which is provided by palliative care trained specialist physicians, typically in a specialty clinic or hospital setting, and involving an interdisciplinary team. Specialty palliative care involves managing complex or refractory symptoms and facilitating communication in challenging situations.[10]

Primary palliative care skills derive from multiple core competencies emphasized by the ACGME for graduating residents in multiple residency programs—internal medicine, family medicine, pediatrics, and others—which emphasize patient-centered communication and aligning treatment plans with patients' goals (components of "interpersonal and communication skills") and basic symptom management ("medical knowledge" and "patient care").[11] Additional programs exist to target subspecialists in multiple areas to learn and practice basic palliative care skills, such as OncoTalk.[12]

In the primary care setting, utilizing these skills for all basic symptom management and psychosocial support without referral to specialist palliative care can strengthen existing relationships between PCPs and their long-term patients and avoid fragmentation of care.

Objectives for Palliative Care in the Primary Care Setting

PCPs are often the first physician that patients encounter as they navigate early stages of a serious illness and are the backbone of a patient's medical care team moving forward. In this way, they are in a unique position to identify patients who need palliative care services, either from themselves or from specialty palliative care providers, and make referrals when indicated. In addition, they may be the only physician that patients see routinely, and through their well-established relationships (often over years), PCPs have the added ability to provide primary palliative care at the same time as providing life-prolonging interventions for chronic conditions.

In the primary care clinic, primary palliative care evaluation can include symptom assessments (including psychological symptoms such as depression or distress) and assisting with advance care planning (ACP). Examples of symptom assessment tools (which can be provided to patients in the office) can be found in **Table 1**, and common symptoms to review will be further explored in the next section. ACP can be guided by many different conversation toolkits currently in existence and designed for use in the primary care setting, such as The Conversation Starter Guide, Serious Illness Conversation Guide, and 5 Wishes, among others.[13–15] We encourage PCPs to engage in conversations about ACP with all patients at some point in their care, prioritizing those with life-limiting illnesses or at advanced age (as recommended by the American Geriatrics Society), in order to increase the likelihood that care will reflect personal preferences of each patient (goal-concordant care).[16,17] For patients with life-limiting illnesses, changes in the disease stage can trigger further discussion about decision-making: when disease worsens, prognosis changes, after hospitalizations, or with decline in performance status. We recommend primary care providers keep copies of advance directives that may exist, including the identification of a medical decision-maker (also known as a health care power of attorney) who would act on behalf of a patient's wishes if necessary.

PRIMARY PALLIATIVE CARE SKILLS
Symptom-Based Management

Patients who are suffering often see their PCP first for symptom management. Therefore, PCPs should have a basic symptom assessment algorithm and treatment toolkit to adequately initiate management and control for their patients. Common chief complaints that PCPs will encounter include chronic pain, constipation, nausea/vomiting, and depression or mood dysregulation. PCPs should become familiar with symptom assessment tools, some of which are found in **Table 1**, which can help with the identification and severity of various symptoms.

Table 1
Common symptom assessment tools for use in the outpatient setting

Symptom Assessment Tools	
Edmonton Symptom Assessment System[87]	9 symptoms assessed, primary for patients with cancer, with rating of severity at time of assessment
Condensed Memorial Symptom Assessment Scale[88]	14 symptoms reviewed and assessed for presence/absence and how bothersome on a scale of 0–4
Brief Pain Inventory[89]	Available in short form (9 questions) and long form (17 questions) and assesses characteristics of pain

Chronic pain is one of the most common reasons why patients seek medical care, either through the Emergency Department or through their primary care providers, and approximately 20% of the US population identifies as having chronic pain.[18,19] Not only does chronic pain cause suffering but it also can limit significant function and mobility for individual patients.[20] Nonpharmacologic therapy and nonopioid pharmacologic agents are first line for treatment of chronic pain, regardless of the cause.[21] Nonpharmacologic therapies that PCPs may recommend include physical therapy, heat or ice therapy, acupuncture, or massage therapy.[22] Pharmacologic treatment should begin by a detailed assessment to differentiate whether the patient is experiencing nociceptive versus neuropathic pain. First-line pharmacologic options for nociceptive pain often include both topical and systemic nonsteroidal anti-inflammatory medications (NSAIDs) and acetaminophen.[23,24] NSAIDs should be used with caution, especially in the geriatric population, given their significant side effect profile, particularly gastrointestinal and cardiovascular toxicity (reviewed in **Table 2**).[25] Nephrotoxic effects are considered rarer, although they should be considered before prescribing.[26]

First-line treatments for neuropathic pain include the gabapentinoids, such as gabapentin and pregabalin, and antidepressants, including medications from serotonin and norepinephrine reuptake inhibitor (SNRI) class and tricyclic antidepressant (TCA) class.[24] In general, SNRIs, such as duloxetine, are preferred over TCAs due to decreased side effect profile.

For severe refractory chronic pain, PCPs can consider opioid therapy. In general, opioids are not recommended for noncancer related chronic pain, and as such, must be used judiciously.[27] If opioids are indicated, prescribers should start with immediate release formulations at the lowest effective dose.[28]

Depression or anxiety is also a chief complaint for many patients encountering their primary care provider. The patient health questionnaire-2 is a screening tool with high sensitivity and low time burden.[29] First-line treatment of depression and anxiety in patients with serious illness follow primary care guidelines of initiating a selective serotonin reuptake inhibitor or SNRI.[30]

Other common complaints include constipation, nausea/vomiting, and fatigue. For many providers, first line management of constipation is typically once or twice daily

Table 2
Review of nonsteroidal anti-inflammatory medication doses and toxicity profile

NSAID Dose and Toxicity Profile		
Medication	**Recommended Dose**	**Toxicity Profile**
Ketorolac	15–30 mg every 6 h for a maximum duration of 5 d	↑↑GI toxicity ↓Cardiovascular toxicity
Aspirin	325–1000 mg every 4–6 h as needed	↑GI toxicity ↓Cardiovascular toxicity
Naproxen	250–500 mg every 12 h as needed	↑GI toxicity ↓Cardiovascular toxicity
Ibuprofen[a]	200–400 mg every 4–6 h as needed OR 600 mg every 6–8 h as needed	Nonselective Mild GI and Cardiovascular toxicities
Celecoxib[a]	100 mg twice daily, maximum dose 400 mg/d	↑Cardiovascular toxicity ↓GI toxicity

[a] Preferred agents due to decreased side effect profile and onset of action.
Data from Qureshi O, Dua. A. COX Inhibitors. In: Publishing S, ed. StatPearls [Internet]. Treasure Island, FL2022.

senna and as needed polyethylene glycol.[31] Patient with nausea and vomiting have many different treatment options but often benefit from metoclopramide or dopamine antagonists such as olanzapine or haloperidol.[32] Fatigue can be difficult to manage but can respond well to lifestyle interventions (such as sleep hygiene training for contributing insomnia or aerobic exercise for cancer-related fatigue) as well as some complementary supplements—American ginseng in particular has been shown to be beneficial for cancer-related fatigue compared with a placebo.[33]

Spiritual Assessment

A key component of palliative care is assessing both the physical, emotional, and spiritual needs of the patient, and often palliative care teams rely on the interdisciplinary team including social workers and chaplains to aid in assessing spiritual health. When integrated with the medical team, receiving spiritual support was associated with 5-fold increased rate of hospice use, as well as fewer aggressive interventions, and ICU deaths.[34] Palliative care team members often utilize spiritual assessment screening tools, several of which are shown in **Table 3**.[35]

Advanced Care Planning

Advanced care planning is a series of conversations between a patient and their medical provider, which involve learning about serious illness and understanding the decisions that may need to be made in the future.[36] These conversations also involve the clinician understanding the goals and wishes of the patient and their family in order to guide patients on their decision-making processes, also known as shared decision-making. Shared decision-making relies on good physician–patient communication and an emphasis on informed consent and autonomy.[37] Physicians therefore not only have the obligation to understand the goals of their patients but also must have a good understanding of the disease process, trajectory, and prognosis.

The primary care clinician and patient relationship already often has the rapport necessary for ACP but clinicians are uncomfortable discussing death and dying. In fact, only 7% of patients discuss their end-of-life wishes with the general practitioner, and only 50% of patients have filled out an advance directive.[38,39] PCPs are primarily worried about destroying patients' hopes, although studies show that patients want to discuss these issues with their trusted providers.[40] Data also show that most Americans prefer to die at home peacefully, the majority end up dying in the hospital setting undergoing aggressive measures.[41]

Advanced care planning and discussions about dying in the outpatient setting can improve end-of-life planning and outcomes.[42] In order to effectively engage with patients on these difficult topics, clinicians must be able to discuss prognosis comfortably and accurately. Studies show that clinicians tend to be overly optimistic when

Table 3 Common spiritual assessment tools for use in the outpatient setting	
Spiritual Assessment Tools	
FICA Spiritual History Tool	Faith and belief, importance, community, address in care
HOPE	Sources of hope, organized religion, personal spirituality and practices, effects on medical care and end-of-life issues
Open Invite Pneumonic	Open the conversation, invite the patient to discuss spiritual needs

Data from Saguil A, Phelps K. The spiritual assessment. *Am Fam Physician.* 2012;86(6):546 to 550.

discussing prognosis,[43] and patients often overestimate the effects of palliative therapy.[44] Inaccurate prognostication can lead to underutilization of hospice services, continuation of potentially harmful screenings, and poorer patient outcomes.[42] However, physicians are deficient at accurately estimating survival,[45] and often, patients have comorbid conditions that can lead to uncertainty in prognosis. One study showed that 87% surrogate decision-makers prefer clinicians to express uncertainty rather than avoid the discussion entirely.[46] Despite patient and surrogate preferences, physicians often do not discuss prognosis, even during serious conversations such as code status discussions, despite the heavy implication on the success of resuscitative efforts.[47]

Several prognostic indicators have been developed in order to aid general practitioners with prognosis, although many of these indices are limited in scope.[48,49] One tool widely used by palliative care providers is ePrognosis (https://eprognosis.ucsf.edu/), which enables users to input a number of different variables and will provide an estimate of prognosis.[50]

Clinicians not only have discomfort with discussions of prognosis and death and dying but they often have discomfort providing recommendations of the care plan based on patient wishes. In the American medical system, clinicians rely heavily on the bioethical principle of autonomy. Many clinicians fear that providing an explicit recommendation will interfere with the autonomous decision-making of the patient. However, in order to effectively allow for autonomous decision-making, providers have the ethical obligation to provide recommendations to their patients founded on knowledge of the disease process and the goals of their patient.[51] In fact, one study demonstrated that a majority of respondents (56%) preferred a recommendation from their provider, compared with 42% who did not want a recommendation.[52] This variation also demonstrates that physicians need to clarify with patients how they wish to receive information and whether or not they wish to receive a recommendation.[42]

Serious Illness Conversation Guide

Appropriately setting up and executing the conversation can be a challenging and important component of ACP discussion. One frequently utilized tool is the *Serious Illness Conversation Guide*, developed by Ariadne laboratories from patient tested language and best practices in palliative care.[53,54] This tool is designed to be printed and utilized during conversations in order to guide clinicians on how to both deliver difficult news but also elicit goals and values from the patient. The recommendations in this guide mirror the techniques used by palliative care physicians.[55] In general, the first step is to ensure an appropriate setting or private environment that will minimize interruptions during the conversation as well as including all members of the family that will be important for decision-making. The next step is to elicit the understanding of the patient and their family on disease process before delivering the prognosis or diagnosis. During this step, it will be important to respond to the emotional reaction of the patient or their family and provide support and empathy. The NURSE pneumonic is a helpful tool to aid in empathic statements (**Table 4**).[56] For these conversations to be successful, clinicians must be empathic and nonjudgmental, as well as allow more time for the patient to speak compared with the physician. One study revealed that clinicians trained in communication emphasized rapport building over information sharing and allowed for twice as much time listening compared with clinicians not trained in communication.[57]

Once these conversations have been initiated, it is important for the physician to protect their patient's wishes. To do so, there are several forms that patients can

Table 4	
NURSE mnemonic for empathic statements	
	NURSE Mnemonic Adapted from VitalTalk
	Example statement
Naming	"I can see how sad this makes you."
Understanding	"This helps me understand where you are coming from."
Respecting	"I can see how hard you have been trying to take care of yourself."
Supporting	"I will do my best to help you throughout this process."
Exploring	"Could you tell me more about..."

Data from Responding to Emotion: Respecting. VitalTalk. VITALtalk Web site. https://www. vitaltalk.org/guides/responding-to-emotion-respecting/. Published 2022. Accessed December 8, 2022.

complete, including an advance directive, which varies based on state as well as Medical Order for Life Sustaining Therapies and Physician Order for Life Sustaining Therapies.[58] Although these documents have legal and ethical implications, ACP is a fluid conversation, and patients and families can always change their minds. In this regard, it is important for clinicians to continue to hold these conversations frequently to assess whether goals and values have shifted.[59]

WHEN TO REFER TO SPECIALTY PALLIATIVE CARE SERVICES?

Recent studies have shown that when serious illness care includes multidisciplinary specialty palliative care, patients have higher quality of life, better outcomes of care, and perhaps even live longer.[1] Both patients and health-care professionals often mistakenly equate palliative care with hospice or end-of-life care and often refer patients late in their disease course. As noted above, palliative care can be used at any time after the diagnosis of a chronic complex or life-limiting illness and services may be delivered concurrently with curative or life-prolonging therapies. The literature shows a clear benefit from early palliative care referral for patients with advanced cancer, and integration of specialty palliative care early in the course of a serious illness is recommended to help manage the physical, psychological, and psychosocial needs of patients.[1,60–62]

Referral in the Outpatient Setting

The benefits of palliative care for patients with a serious illness are maximized through early integration in the illness trajectory and the outpatient setting is ideal for this care. A variety of models exist for outpatient palliative care, including stand-alone clinics, embedded clinics, telehealth-based palliative care, and advanced practice provider-enhanced primary palliative care.[63] Current literature has mostly examined stand-alone clinics in which care is delivered by an interdisciplinary specialist palliative care team and has confirmed the benefits of early palliative care referral in this setting.[63]

Embedded clinics are a common variation of outpatient palliative care in which palliative care team members are embedded in the primary office, usually the oncology clinic. This model has both advantages and disadvantages but there is a paucity of literature regarding this model.[64] Telehealth palliative care may be used to supplement traditional outpatient visits and is also used for managing patients who live in remote or underserved areas.[65] Telehealth palliative care also remains an underresearched area. Enhanced primary care, the practice of providing a trained advanced practice provider in the specialty clinic, has not been shown to result in improved patient outcomes.[66]

In the outpatient setting, the most common activities that palliative care clinicians engage in include introducing the concept of palliative care, managing symptoms, supporting families, coordinating care, and helping patients understand their illness, prognosis, and treatment options.[67]

Community-based palliative care programs represent an additional type of outpatient setting and provide interdisciplinary support for patients with serious illness at home or community-based care facilities such as postacute and long-term care facilities. Home-based palliative care has been shown to improve symptom control and increase the rate of home death.[63] As is the case for outpatient palliative care, earlier involvement in community-based palliative care is associated with better outcomes.[68]

When to Consider Hospice Referral?

Hospice is a philosophy of care that focuses on patients who have a life expectancy of less than 6 months and is focused on comfort rather than cure or prolongation of life. Although it is an important component of palliative care, the terms are not interchangeable. Referral should be made when the patient has a prognosis of less than or equal to 6 months, and it is consistent with their goals. Hospice care is associated with better symptom relief, patient-goal attainment, and quality of end-of-life care, particularly if they are referred earlier in their disease trajectory.[69] Referral is often delayed for multiple reasons including prognostic uncertainty and discomfort talking about death.[70] As noted previously, here are validated tools to aid clinicians in determining prognosis for patients with and without cancer[70-74] as well as structured communication strategies designed to make hospice discussions more effective.[75] Explicit and clear communication regarding what hospice care entails is key in order to avoid misunderstanding on the patient's part.

Hospice services are provided by an interdisciplinary team, usually consisting of a nurse, social worker, home health aides, chaplain, volunteers, and the physician hospice medical director. In the United States, the Medicare Hospice Benefit (MHB) pays for 80% of all hospice care. Medicaid and private insurance also cover hospice services.[76] To enroll in the MHB, the patient must be certified by the Hospice Medical Director and the primary physician as having a life expectancy of less than 6 months. Patients can continue to be eligible if they live longer than 6 months if the physicians think death will likely occur within 6 months. The MHB provides 4 levels of care: routine home care, general inpatient care, continuous care, and respite care. Most hospice care is routine home care. The MHB covers durable medical equipment, the cost of all medications related to the hospice diagnosis, 24-hour, 7-day telephone access to a hospice provider, usually a nurse, and in-person access to a hospice provider when needed. The general inpatient benefit covers patients who need to be hospitalized or admitted to an inpatient hospice facility to control symptoms, while the continuous care benefit covers between 8 and 24 hours of medical care in the patient's home if needed. The MHB also provides up to 5 days of respite care in a facility.

PALLIATIVE CARE MANAGEMENT OF PATIENTS WITH HIGH-RISK OPIATE USE
Opioid Use Disorder and Opioid Misuse in Patients with Cancer and Cancer Survivors

Pain related to advanced cancer is common, and opioid pain medications remain an essential component of pain management in these patients.[77] That said, it is clear that opioids can cause harm, including unintentional overdose and death, and patients with cancer and cancer survivors have similar rates of opioid use disorder (OUD) as other populations as well as a high rate of opioid misuse.[78] Additionally, untreated substance use disorders can complicate the treatment of pain. Because primary care clinicians play an important role in primary palliative care, it is important to have an understanding of safe opioid prescribing as well as recognition and management of opioid misuse and OUD in this population.

Currently, the universal precaution approach to prescribing opioids is recommended for patients with cancer pain. This approach, which is based on evidence from the non-cancer population,[79] involves appropriate pain assessment, screening for risk of developing OUD, informed consent, treatment agreement, use of nonopioid and nonpharmacologic pain management strategies, monitoring for risk, and regular follow-up. **Table 5** presents a summary of the universal precaution prescribing method.

If the initial risk is high, or if patients demonstrate behaviors consistent with opioid misuse, more frequent monitoring, including urine drug tests (UDTs), is indicated. Clinicians should have open communication with patients[80] who demonstrate opioid

Table 5
Summary of universal prescribing precautions for chronic opioid therapy in patients with cancer

Step	Precaution	Explanation
1	Complete Pain Assessment	Make an appropriate diagnosis of pain, type and review effective therapies
2	Consideration of appropriate nonopioid and nonpharmacological treatments	
3	Initial screening	Risk assessment tools include: • Opioid Risk Tool[90] • Screener and Opioid Assessment for Patients with Pain (SOAPP)[91]; Revised Screener and Opioid Assessment (SOAPP-R)[92]
4	Discuss risks and benefits of opioid pain management and obtain informed consent	Obtain consent through a written treatment agreement that outlines risks, benefits of opioid pain medicine, patient's and physician's responsibilities. Provide education on safe use, storage, and disposal
5	Employ risk mitigation strategies	• Regular follow-up appointments are important to determine treatment efficacy and to reevaluate benefits and risks of continued therapy • Check the state prescription drug monitoring program before each opioid prescription, and UDT periodically and use results to determine treatment adherence and assess risks of the opioid pain medicine
6	Avoid concurrent benzodiazepine prescriptions	
7	If risks outweigh benefits of opioid pain management, consider referral to interdisciplinary specialty palliative care and/or addiction medicine specialist	

Data from: Dowell D, Ragan KR, Jones CM, Baldwin GT, Chou R. CDC Clinical Practice Guideline for Prescribing Opioids for Pain-United States, 2022. MMWR Recomm Rep. 2022 Nov 4;71(3):1-95

misuse including the implications, which may include more frequent visits, limited opioid quantity, and more frequent monitoring. Increased behavioral health support may also benefit these patients.

Advanced patients with cancer who develop or have preexisting OUD[81] can be challenging to manage but treatment of both OUD and severe pain is essential. Strategies include using buprenorphine or methadone for treatment of both pain and OUD.[82] Interdisciplinary specialty palliative care can be very useful in managing these patients and can be another support for the PCP.

In cancer survivors with chronic pain, consideration should be given to a patient-centered taper. This should include supportive, shared decision-making, and sudden discontinuing or rapid taper is rarely indicated.[83] In cancer survivors with OUD, office-based rotation to buprenorphine should be offered.

An increasing number of people are being treated with medications to treat opioid use disorder (MOUD) including buprenorphine and methadone. Expert opinion consensus on how to manage pain in cancer patients with OUD including those treated with MOUD has been recently published.[84,85]

It is important to understand that all physicians can prescribe both buprenorphine and methadone for pain management. To prescribe buprenorphine for OUD, a federal Drug Enforcement Agency X-waiver is no longer required, and however methadone must be prescribed in a federally regulated opioid treatment program. Relatively few primary and palliative care physicians have X-waivers and barriers to prescribing buprenorphine for both pain and OUD. However, with the elimination of the X-waiver and pain management preparation of these medications, the impact on primary care provider using these medications will need to be further explored.[86] Buprenorphine is a preferred medication in the elderly because it can be used on patient with renal impairment and has a greater margin of safety.

Finally, it is essential for all physicians to embrace harm reduction. All patients prescribed greater than 50 mg oral morphine equivalents should receive a prescription for naloxone as should all patients with OUD.

SUMMARY

Palliative care is no longer synonymous with end-of-life care, and as supply has been well outstripped by demand, much of the practice of palliative care early in a patient's illness journey will take place in the primary care clinic—referred to as primary palliative care. Primary palliative care skills, including symptom and spiritual assessments, as well as basic ACP conversations, are essential for caring for older adults and a key component in the education and training of internists and geriatricians. Referral to specialty palliative care for complex symptom management or clarification on decision-making is appropriate as an additional layer of support for patients and PCPs. Knowing when to refer patients for specialty palliative care and hospice, if indicated, is critical in maximizing patients' quality of life throughout their entire disease course, and benefits both patients and caregivers.

CLINICS CARE POINTS

- Primary palliative care is a necessary component of outpatient practice and includes symptom management skills, such as utilization of symptom assessment tools, and advance care planning.
- Toolkits such as the Serious Illness Conversation Guide can be helpful to begin ACP discussions in the outpatient primary care setting.

- Universal precaution should be used when prescribing opiates for cancer pain, including pain assessment, screening for risk of developing OUD, informed consent, and use of adjuvant non-opioid and non-pharmacologic pain management strategies, as well as regular follow up for risk monitoring.

DISCLOSURE

There are no financial or commercial conflicts of interest for any authors.

REFERENCES

1. Temel JS, Greer JA, Muzikansky A, et al. Early palliative care for patients with metastatic non–small-cell lung cancer. N Engl J Med 2010;363(8):733–42.
2. Smith TJ, Temin S, Alesi ER, et al. American society of clinical oncology provisional clinical opinion: the integration of palliative care into standard oncology care. J Clin Oncol 2012;30(8):880–7.
3. Medicine AAoHaP. Program Data. Available at: http://aahpm.org/uploads/Program_Data_102820.pdf. Published 2021. Accessed November 18, 2022, 2022.
4. Center HaPC. HPCC History. Available at: https://advancingexpertcare.org/HPCC/About_Us/History.aspx. Published 2012. Accessed November 18, 2022.
5. Workers NAoS. Advanced Certified Hospice and Palliative Social Worker (ACHP-SW). Available at: https://www.socialworkers.org/careers/credentials-certifications/apply-for-nasw-social-work-credentials/advanced-certified-hospice-and-palliative-social-worker. Published 2022. Accessed November 18, 2022, 2022.
6. Board of Chaplaincy Certification I. Available at: https://bcci.professionalchaplains.org/content.asp?contentid=45. Published 2020. Accessed November 18, 2022, 2022.
7. Care CtAP. Growth of Palliative Care in US Hospitals - 2022 Snapshot. Available at: https://www.capc.org/documents/download/1031/. Published 2022. Accessed November 18, 2022, 2022.
8. Care CtAP. Report Card. https://reportcard.capc.org/. Published 2019. Accessed November 18, 2022, 2022.
9. Kamal AH, Bull JH, Swetz KM, et al. Future of the palliative care workforce: preview to an impending crisis. Am J Med 2017;130(2):113–4.
10. Quill TE, Abernethy AP. Generalist plus specialist palliative care–creating a more sustainable model. N Engl J Med 2013;368(13):1173–5.
11. Education ACfGM. Implementing milestones and clinical competency committees. Available at: http://www.acgme.org/acgmeweb/Portals/0/PDFs/ACGME Milestones-CCC-AssesmentWebinar.pdf. Accessed November 28, 2022, 2022.
12. Back AL, Arnold RM, Baile WF, et al. Faculty development to change the paradigm of communication skills teaching in oncology. J Clin Oncol: official journal of the American Society of Clinical Oncology 2009;27(7):1137.
13. Improvement IfH. The Conversation Starter Guide. Available at: https://theconversationproject.org/wp-content/uploads/2020/12/ConversationStarter Guide.pdf. Published 2022. Accessed November 28, 2022, 2022.
14. Labs A. Serious Illness Conversation Guide. Available at: https://www.ariadnelabs.org/wp-content/uploads/2017/05/SI-CG-2017-04-21_FINAL.pdf. Published 2015. Accessed November 28, 2022, 2022.
15. Dignity Aw. Five Wishes. Available at: https://www.fivewishes.org/. Published 2022. Accessed November 28, 2022, 2022.

16. Society AG. Advance Care Planning for Older Adults. Available at: https://www.americangeriatrics.org/sites/default/files/inline-files/AGS%20Statement%20on%20Advance%20Care%20Planning_FINAL%20%28August%202017%29.pdf. Published 2017. Accessed November 28, 2022, 2022.

17. Detering KM, Hancock AD, Reade MC, et al. The impact of advance care planning on end of life care in elderly patients: randomised controlled trial. BMJ 2010; 340:c1345.

18. Schappert SM, Burt CW. Ambulatory care visits to physician offices, hospital outpatient departments, and emergency departments: United States, 2001-02. Vital Health Stat 2006;13(159):1–66.

19. Dahlhamer J, Lucas J, Zelaya C, et al. Prevalence of chronic pain and high-impact chronic pain among adults - United States, 2016. MMWR Morb Mortal Wkly Rep 2018;67(36):1001–6.

20. Gureje O, Von Korff M, Simon GE, et al. Persistent pain and well-being: a world health organization study in primary care. JAMA 1998;280(2):147–51.

21. Centers For Disease C, Prevention Public Health Service USDOH, Human S. Guideline for prescribing opioids for chronic pain. J Pain Palliat Care Pharmacother 2016;30(2):138–40.

22. Adams ML, Arminio GJ. Non-pharmacologic pain management intervention. Clin Podiatr Med Surg 2008;25(3):409–29, vi.

23. Ferrell B, Argoff CE, Epplin J, et al. Pharmacological management of persistent pain in older persons. J Am Geriatr Soc 2009;57(8):1331–46.

24. Gloth FM 3rd. Pharmacological management of persistent pain in older persons: focus on opioids and nonopioids. J Pain 2011;12(3 Suppl 1):S14–20.

25. Qureshi O. and Dua A., COX inhibitors, In: StatPearls [internet], 2023, Treasure Island; FL. Available at: https://www.ncbi.nlm.nih.gov/books/NBK549795/.

26. Wongrakpanich S, Wongrakpanich A, Melhado K, et al. A comprehensive review of non-steroidal anti-inflammatory drug use in the elderly. Aging Dis 2018;9(1): 143–50.

27. Chou R, Turner JA, Devine EB, et al. The effectiveness and risks of long-term opioid therapy for chronic pain: a systematic review for a National Institutes of Health Pathways to Prevention Workshop. Ann Intern Med 2015;162(4):276–86.

28. Pharmacologic management of chronic non-cancer pain in adults, 2022, Wolters Kluwer, Available at: https://www.uptodate.com/contents/pharmacologic-management-of-chronic-non-cancer-pain-in-adults. Accessed December 8, 2022.

29. Levis B, Sun Y, He C, et al. Accuracy of the PHQ-2 alone and in combination with the PHQ-9 for screening to detect major depression: systematic review and meta-analysis. JAMA 2020;323(22):2290–300.

30. Gautam S, Jain A, Gautam M, et al. Clinical practice guidelines for the management of depression. Indian J Psychiatry 2017;59(Suppl 1):S34–50.

31. Portalatin M, Winstead N. Medical management of constipation. Clin Colon Rectal Surg 2012;25(1):12–9.

32. Gupta M, Davis M, LeGrand S, et al. Nausea and vomiting in advanced cancer: the Cleveland Clinic protocol. J Support Oncol 2013;11(1):8–13.

33. Barton DL, Liu H, Dakhil SR, et al. Wisconsin Ginseng (Panax quinquefolius) to improve cancer-related fatigue: a randomized, double-blind trial, N07C2. J Natl Cancer Inst 2013;105(16):1230–8.

34. Balboni TA, Balboni M, Enzinger AC, et al. Provision of spiritual support to patients with advanced cancer by religious communities and associations with medical care at the end of life. JAMA Intern Med 2013;173(12):1109–17.

35. Saguil A, Phelps K. The spiritual assessment. Am Fam Physician 2012;86(6): 546–50.
36. *Advance care planning: health care directives*, 2018, National Institutes of Health, Washington, DC, Available at: https://www.nia.nih.gov/health/advance-care-planning-advance-directives-health-care. Accessed December 8, 2022.
37. Elwyn G, Frosch D, Thomson R, et al. Shared decision making: a model for clinical practice. J Gen Intern Med 2012;27(10):1361–7.
38. Solis GR, Mancera BM, Shen MJ. Strategies used to facilitate the discussion of advance care planning with older adults in primary care settings: a literature review. J Am Assoc Nurse Pract 2018;30(5):270–9.
39. Benson W, Aldrich N. Advance care planning: ensuring your wishes are known and honored if you are unable to speak for yourself, 2012 you are unable to speak for yourself, critical issue brief. Decatur, GA: Centers for Disease Control and Prevention; 2012.
40. Murray SA, Sheikh A, Thomas K. Advance care planning in primary care. BMJ 2006;333(7574):868–9.
41. IOM (Institute of Medicine). 2015. Dying in America: Improving quality and honoring individual preferences near the end of life. Washington, DC: The National Academies Press. 1, Introduction. Available at: https://www.ncbi.nlm.nih.gov/books/NBK285681/.
42. Ghosh A, Dzeng E, Cheng MJ. Interaction of palliative care and primary care. Clin Geriatr Med 2015;31(2):207–18.
43. Christakis NA, Lamont EB. Extent and determinants of error in doctors' prognoses in terminally ill patients: prospective cohort study. BMJ 2000;320(7233):469–72.
44. Weeks JC, Catalano PJ, Cronin A, et al. Patients' expectations about effects of chemotherapy for advanced cancer. N Engl J Med 2012;367(17):1616–25.
45. Warraich HJ, Allen LA, Mukamal KJ, et al. Accuracy of physician prognosis in heart failure and lung cancer: comparison between physician estimates and model predicted survival. Palliat Med 2016;30(7):684–9.
46. Evans LR, Boyd EA, Malvar G, et al. Surrogate decision-makers' perspectives on discussing prognosis in the face of uncertainty. Am J Respir Crit Care Med 2009; 179(1):48–53.
47. Anderson WG, Chase R, Pantilat SZ, et al. Code status discussions between attending hospitalist physicians and medical patients at hospital admission. J Gen Intern Med 2011;26(4):359–66.
48. Yourman LC, Lee SJ, Schonberg MA, et al. Prognostic indices for older adults: a systematic review. JAMA 2012;307(2):182–92.
49. Walter LC, Brand RJ, Counsell SR, et al. Development and validation of a prognostic index for 1-year mortality in older adults after hospitalization. JAMA 2001;285(23):2987–94.
50. ePrognosis|Calculators. University of California San Francisco. Available at: https://eprognosis.ucsf.edu/calculators/index.php. Accessed December 8, 2022.
51. Guidelines for the appropriate use of do-not-resuscitate orders. Council on ethical and judicial affairs, American medical association. JAMA 1991;265(14): 1868–71.
52. White DB, Evans LR, Bautista CA, et al. Are physicians' recommendations to limit life support beneficial or burdensome? Bringing empirical data to the debate. Am J Respir Crit Care Med 2009;180(4):320–5.
53. Bernacki R, Hutchings M, Vick J, et al. Development of the Serious Illness Care Program: a randomised controlled trial of a palliative care communication intervention. BMJ Open 2015;5(10):e009032.

54. Labs A. Serious Illness Conversation Guide. Ariadne Labs. Tolls for Clinicians Web site. Available at: https://www.ariadnelabs.org/serious-illness-care/for-clinicians/. Published 2022. Accessed December 8, 2022.
55. Rosenzweig MQ. Breaking bad news: a guide for effective and empathetic communication. Nurse Pract 2012;37(2):1–4.
56. Responding to Emotion: Respecting. VitalTalk. VITALtalk Web site. Available at: https://www.vitaltalk.org/guides/responding-to-emotion-respecting/. Published 2022. Accessed December 8, 2022.
57. Roter DL, Larson S, Fischer GS, et al. Experts practice what they preach: a descriptive study of best and normative practices in end-of-life discussions. Arch Intern Med 2000;160(22):3477–85.
58. Meier DE, Beresford L. POLST offers next stage in honoring patient preferences. J Palliat Med 2009;12(4):291–5.
59. Tulsky JA. Beyond advance directives: importance of communication skills at the end of life. JAMA 2005;294(3):359–65.
60. Ferrell BR, Temel JS, Temin S, et al. Integration of palliative care into standard oncology care: American society of clinical oncology clinical practice guideline update. J Clin Oncol 2017;35(1):96–112.
61. Greer JA, Pirl WF, Jackson VA, et al. Effect of early palliative care on chemotherapy use and end-of-life care in patients with metastatic non-small-cell lung cancer. J Clin Oncol 2012;30(4):394–400.
62. Temel JS, Greer JA, Admane S, et al. Longitudinal perceptions of prognosis and goals of therapy in patients with metastatic non-small-cell lung cancer: results of a randomized study of early palliative care. J Clin Oncol 2011;29(17):2319–26.
63. Hui D, Bruera E. Models of palliative care delivery for patients with cancer. J Clin Oncol 2020;38(9):852–65.
64. Hui D, Bruera E. Models of integration of oncology and palliative care. Ann Palliat Med 2015;4(3):89–98.
65. Gordon B, Mason B, Smith SLH. Leveraging telehealth for delivery of palliative care to remote communities: a rapid review. J Palliat Care 2022;37(2):213–25.
66. Hui D. Palliative cancer care in the outpatient setting: which model works best? Curr Treat Options Oncol 2019;20(2):17.
67. Bischoff K, Yang E, Kojimoto G, et al. What we do: key activities of an outpatient palliative care team at an academic cancer center. J Palliat Med 2018;21(7):999–1004.
68. Pellizzari M, Hui D, Pinato E, et al. Impact of intensity and timing of integrated home palliative cancer care on end-of-life hospitalization in Northern Italy. Support Care Cancer 2017;25(4):1201–7.
69. Kumar P, Wright AA, Hatfield LA, et al. Family perspectives on hospice care experiences of patients with cancer. J Clin Oncol 2017;35(4):432–9.
70. Greenstein JE, Policzer JS, Shaban ES. Hospice for the primary care physician. Prim Care 2019;46(3):303–17.
71. Levy WC, Mozaffarian D, Linker DT, et al. The Seattle Heart Failure Model: prediction of survival in heart failure. Circulation 2006;113(11):1424–33.
72. Celli BR, Cote CG, Marin JM, et al. The body-mass index, airflow obstruction, dyspnea, and exercise capacity index in chronic obstructive pulmonary disease. N Engl J Med 2004;350(10):1005–12.
73. Said A, Williams J, Holden J, et al. Model for end stage liver disease score predicts mortality across a broad spectrum of liver disease. J Hepatol 2004;40(6):897–903.

74. Beddhu S, Bruns FJ, Saul M, et al. A simple comorbidity scale predicts clinical outcomes and costs in dialysis patients. Am J Med 2000;108(8):609–13.
75. Casarett DJ, Quill TE. "I'm not ready for hospice": strategies for timely and effective hospice discussions. Ann Intern Med 2007;146(6):443–9.
76. Center for Medicaid and Medicare Services. Medicare Benefit Policy Manual: Chaper 9: Coverage of Hospice Services Under Hospital Insurance. 2021. Available at: https://www.cms.gov/Regulations-and-Guidance/Guidance/Manuals/Downloads/bp102c09.pdf. Accessed May 2, 2023.
77. Paice JA. Under pressure: the tension between access and abuse of opioids in cancer pain management. J Oncol Pract 2017;13(9):595–6.
78. Preux C, Bertin M, Tarot A, et al. Prevalence of opioid use disorder among patients with cancer-related pain: a systematic review. J Clin Med 2022;11(6):1594.
79. Dowell D, Ragan KR, Jones CM, et al. CDC clinical practice guideline for prescribing opioids for pain - United States, 2022. MMWR Recomm Rep (Morb Mortal Wkly Rep) 2022;71(3):1–95.
80. Sager Z, Childers J. Navigating challenging conversations about nonmedical opioid use in the context of oncology. Oncol 2019;24(10):1299–304.
81. Diagnostic and statistical manual of mental disorders. Washington DCAPA: DSM-5; 2013.
82. Case AA, Kullgren J, Anwar S, et al. Treating chronic pain with buprenorphine-the practical guide. Curr Treat Options Oncol 2021;22(12):116.
83. Jones KF, Merlin JS. Approaches to opioid prescribing in cancer survivors: lessons learned from the general literature. Cancer 2022;128(3):449–55.
84. Fitzgerald Jones K, Khodyakov D, Arnold R, et al. Consensus-based guidance on opioid management in individuals with advanced cancer-related pain and opioid misuse or use disorder. JAMA Oncol 2022;8(8):1107–14.
85. Merlin JS, Khodyakov D, Arnold R, et al. Expert panel consensus on management of advanced cancer-related pain in individuals with opioid use disorder. JAMA Netw Open 2021;4(12):e2139968.
86. Janet Ho J, Jones KF, Sager Z, et al. Barriers to buprenorphine prescribing for opioid use disorder in hospice and palliative care. J Pain Symptom Manage 2022;64(2):119–27.
87. Bruera E, Kuehn N, Miller MJ, et al. The Edmonton Symptom Assessment System (ESAS): a simple method for the assessment of palliative care patients. J Palliat Care 1991;7(2):6–9.
88. Bircan HA, Yalcin GS, Fidanci S, et al. The usefulness and prognostic value of memorial symptom assessment-short form and condensed memorial symptom assessment scale in assessment of lung cancer patients. Support Care Cancer 2020;28(4):2005–14.
89. Daut RL, Cleeland CS, Flanery RC. Development of the Wisconsin Brief Pain Questionnaire to assess pain in cancer and other diseases. Pain 1983;17(2):197–210.
90. Webster LR, Webster RM. Predicting aberrant behaviors in opioid-treated patients: preliminary validation of the Opioid Risk Tool. Pain Med 2005;6(6):432–42.
91. Akbik H, Butler SF, Budman SH, et al. Validation and clinical application of the screener and opioid assessment for patients with pain (SOAPP). J Pain Symptom Manage 2006;32(3):287–93.
92. Butler SF, Fernandez K, Benoit C, et al. Validation of the revised screener and opioid assessment for patients with pain (SOAPP-R). J Pain 2008;9(4):360–72.

Public Health and Palliative Care

Sarah H. Cross, PhD, MSW, MPH*, Dio Kavalieratos, PhD

KEYWORDS

- End of life • Public health • Palliative care • Hospice

KEY POINTS

- Meeting the needs of people at the end of life (EOL) is a public health (PH) concern, yet a PH approach has not been widely applied to EOL care.
- The design of hospice in the United States, with its focus on cost containment, has resulted in disparities in EOL care use and quality.
- Individuals with non-cancer diagnoses, minoritized individuals, individuals of lower socioeconomic status, and those who do not yet qualify for hospice are particularly disadvantaged by the existing hospice policy.
- New models of palliative care (both hospice and non-hospice) are needed to equitably address the burden of suffering from a serious illness.

PALLIATIVE CARE AS A PUBLIC HEALTH PRIORITY

Meeting the needs of older people at the end of life (EOL) is a pressing public health (PH) issue.[1,2] EOL suffering shares the defining characteristics of other PH priorities: large burden, major impact regarding health consequences or costs, and the potential for prevention.[2,3] More than 3 million Americans die annually and most individuals are unlikely to receive the care they need throughout their course of illness.[4,5] Many seriously-ill individuals experience unrelieved physical and psychosocial needs and reports of these distressing symptoms at the EOL are increasing.[6–8] Changing social structures have altered the availability of family caregivers, a vital but often unacknowledged part of the health care system.[9]

Our aging population and associated increased health care costs also pose significant economic challenges. The costs of caring for individuals in their last year of life are estimated to account for 13% of total annual health care spending in the United States.[10] Many individuals are willing to make substantial financial sacrifices to pay

This work was supported by the NIH, United States-funded Georgia CTSA KL2 and UL1 grants (KL2TR002381 and UL1TR002378).
Division of Palliative Medicine, Department of Family and Preventive Medicine, Emory University, 1518 Clifton Road Northeast, Atlanta, GA 30322, USA
* Corresponding author.
E-mail address: shcross@emory.edu

for serious illness treatment.[11] Long-term financial hardships from lost income due to serious illness and difficulties affording medication and food are common.[12,13]

PH has been defined as "the science and art of preventing disease, prolonging life, and promoting health through the organized efforts and informed choices of society, organizations, public and private communities, and individuals."[14] However, health is not merely the absence of disease.[15] Eventually in the course of illness, the goal of care shifts from disease prevention or cure to the minimization of the suffering resulting from disease. Yet to date, the role of PH approaches and systems thinking has not been widely applied to EOL care. Palliative care (PC), including hospice, provides various models by which to improve EOL at the population level.

HOSPICE AS PUBLIC HEALTH PREVENTION

At EOL, the primary method for the prevention and reduction of suffering is hospice. Hospice has been associated with lower rates of hospitalization, intensive care unit (ICU) admission, and invasive procedures at the EOL.[16] It has also been associated with reductions in symptom distress, improved care quality, improved outcomes for caregivers, and high patient and family satisfaction.[17–21] Hospice has also been associated with reduced medical expenditures.[16,19,22]

Total Medicare hospice enrollment in the United States increased from 513,000 to more than 1.7 million beneficiaries between 2000 and 2020.[23] Despite this increase, disparities in hospice utilization persist among individuals with non-cancer diagnoses, minoritized individuals, and those experiencing greater socioeconomic needs. Additionally, seriously ill individuals who do not qualify for hospice often experience unmet needs as non-hospice PC is not widely available. Although the value of a PH approach to serious illness-related suffering has been recognized, EOL care provision remains fragmented and insufficient for many. The development of American hospice, its history, and design, informs the care available today.

HOSPICE AND PALLIATIVE CARE IN THE UNITED STATES

The first modern hospice, St. Christopher's, was opened in London, England, in 1967 by Cicely Saunders and colleagues who were motivated by the neglect of and lack of research on those dying from cancer.[24] Saunders' work inspired the establishment of the first hospice in the United States in 1973. Hospice in the United Kingdom was mostly an inpatient service; however, several factors contributed to American hospice emphasizing home care: a desire for independence, a distrust of medical institutions, and a lack of resources for non-profit hospices operating outside mainstream medicine.[25] As the hospice movement grew, so did professional organizations and the push for hospice reimbursement.[24,25]

In 1980, the Health Care Financing Administration, a precursor to the Centers for Medicare and Medicaid Services, established a demonstration project to examine the impact of hospice on cancer patients' quality of life and health care costs.[26] The 3-year National Hospice Study (NHS) was created to examine the costs and benefits of providing hospice to terminally-ill cancer patients.[26] Although the study eventually found that hospice achieved comparable outcomes to conventional cancer care and was generally less costly, hospice became a Medicare benefit before the NHS was complete.[27]

Medicare Hospice Benefit

Hospice was marketed in congressional hearings as a low-cost Medicare benefit and was included as an amendment to the Tax Equity and Fiscal Responsibility Act

(TEFRA) of 1982 with a 3-year sunset provision before becoming a permanent benefit in 1985.[26] One of TEFRA's cost-saving provisions was that patients signing on to hospice must forgo traditional medical services, creating a substitute for rather than a supplement to traditional care.[25,26]

Data from the NHS showed that hospice costs were greatest at the time of admission and during the last days of life.[28] Hospice was only cost-saving if used for less than 30 days and if associated with fewer days in the hospital at the EOL. If hospice referrals occurred very close to death, hospice was not associated with cost savings. If hospice use began long before the "terminal period" when a patient would typically become hospitalized, hospice costs would exceed the savings in hospital costs. Therefore, achieving cost savings for hospice required a distribution of hospice length of stays that were not too long. For this reason, the initial Medicare hospice benefit (MHB) permitted 210 days of hospice services, which were divided into two initial 90-day eligibility periods and a final 30-day period.[26] These have since been updated to allow for an initial 90-day period, a subsequent 90-day period, followed by an unlimited number of subsequent 60-day periods.[23] Additionally, the legislation also included aggregate payment caps limiting the percentage of a hospice's days that could be inpatient and the average annual per patient costs of hospice's patients. Mor and Teno note that hospice fiscal viability has been dependent upon having a mix of patients, limiting inpatient services and the frequency and length of visits, using lower cost personnel, and relying on family members to provide hands-on care.[26] As a result, hospices may be less likely to accept patients with more costly and complex needs.[29]

DIAGNOSIS-RELATED DISPARITIES AT END OF LIFE

Hospice patients of today are epidemiologically different from the patients for whom the MHB was designed. In the early days of hospice, more than 90% of patients had a primary diagnosis of cancer; however, cancer is no longer the primary diagnosis of most hospice patients.[25,30] This has led to unequal hospice use by patients of different diagnoses and has implications for quality of care at EOL.

Heart Failure

Only about one-third of individuals with heart failure (HF) receive hospice at the time of death.[31] Most individuals with HF that do use hospice tend to enroll late in their disease course, when otherwise preventable suffering has already impacted patients and their families.[32,33] Individuals with HF who enroll in hospice use less health care and are less likely to die in the hospital.[34]

Unlike individuals with cancer, who tend to have a sharp decline in the final months of life, individuals with HF often experience a gradual decline with frequent exacerbations.[35] Following treatment, they may return to near-baseline status[36,37]; however, eventually one of these exacerbations will be fatal and death is often unexpected.[38] This unpredictable trajectory makes prognostication and, therefore, knowing when hospice is appropriate (by statute, not by need), difficult.[39]

Individuals with HF experience a greater symptom severity than individuals with advanced cancer, especially dyspnea, fatigue, and pain.[39–42] Many caregivers of those with HF feel unprepared to deal with exacerbations at home.[43,44] Worsening symptoms and caregiver unpreparedness likely contribute to HF being the leading cause of hospital readmissions in the United States.[45] Hospice use has been associated with a lower risk of 30-day hospital readmission among patients with HF.[46]

Dementia

Several barriers to hospice use among people with dementia have been identified. Perhaps most importantly, dementia has been under-recognized as a terminal illness.[47,48] As recognition of terminal status is essential for both referral to and enrollment in hospice, this fact may place individuals with dementia at risk of receiving suboptimal EOL care.

Dementia has greater variability in survival from diagnosis to death than other hospice diagnoses[49–51] and is often seen as having contributed to a terminal event, rather than as the cause of death itself.[47,48,52,53] The lack of prognostic indicators and variable survival do not fit with a hospice benefit that requires physician certification that an individual has a probable life expectancy of 6 months or less.

Although most individuals with dementia in the United States die in nursing facilities, many residents do not receive the care in hospice.[54] Many people come to a skilled nursing facility (SNF) following a hospitalization. Medicare beneficiaries who have been hospitalized for 3 days and have a skilled need are entitled to 100 days of SNF care. Regulations prevent the use of the MHB concurrent with the use of Medicare's posthospitalization benefit if SNF care is related to the hospice diagnosis. If an SNF resident would like to use the MHB, the SNF room and board must be paid by Medicaid or out of pocket by the resident/family. As facilities receive higher reimbursement under the Medicare SNF benefit than they would from Medicaid for custodial care, it may be financially disadvantageous for patients to enroll in hospice.[55,56]

End-Stage Renal Disease

The inability to receive concurrent hospice and life-extending treatment is uniquely problematic for individuals with end-stage renal disease (ESRD). Unlike hospice patients with cancer who may receive palliative chemotherapy or radiation, Medicare policy prevents receipt of palliative dialysis unless the patient is enrolled in hospice under a diagnosis other than ESRD. Patients undergoing hemodialysis and nearing the EOL must choose between either stopping dialysis and entering hospice or continuing dialysis and forgoing the benefits of hospice.[57] A recent study of hemodialysis patients found that more than 41% entered hospice within the last 3 days of life,[58] meaning they and their families likely do not receive the full benefits that hospice can provide.[59–61]

RACIAL DISPARITIES AT THE END OF LIFE

In 2020, 33.3% of Hispanic Americans, 36.1% of Asian Americans, and 33.5% of Native Americans used hospice compared to 50.8% of White Americans.[23] Near the EOL, Black individuals use emergency services, are on a respirator, and have a feeding tube more often than Whites.[62,63] Although active medical service is increased for Black individuals, the use of hospice is notably lower. This underutilization of hospice has been associated with increased suffering, increased ICU use, increased likelihood of in-hospital death, and higher medical costs.[62,64,65] Black patients are also more likely than White patients to revoke hospice to pursue life-prolonging therapies.[66] Additionally, Black people are more likely than Whites to die in the hospital.[67]

Hispanic Americans are more likely than White Americans to receive life-sustaining treatment at the EOL and to die in the hospital.[64,68,69] Individuals living in census tracts with a greater percentage of Black and Hispanic residents are less likely to use hospice than individuals in areas with fewer minorities, independent of socioeconomic and clinical factors.[70] Language, religious beliefs, and family culture have been identified as barriers to hospice use among Hispanic Americans.[71] Higher education has been associated with greater knowledge about hospice among immigrants from Central and South America.[72]

Asian Americans are more likely to have prolonged frequent hospitalizations, ICU admissions, and to die in the hospital than Whites.[69,73] Asian Americans use hospice less often than White Americans and American-born Asians use hospice more than foreign-born Asians.[74,75] Members of Asian populations have reported low familiarity with hospice and EOL services[76–78] However, more attention is now being paid to the structural inequities and racism that create barriers to use. This is in addition to the benefit of not being flexible enough to meet the needs of minoritized communities at the EOL. Research is moving away from focusing on individual cultural factors as barriers and evaluating inherent environment and institutional barriers to hospice enrollment. Understanding how the diversity of our aging society impacts hospice utilization is important for ensuring that care at EOL is equitable.

SOCIOECONOMIC DISPARITIES AT END OF LIFE

Low-income individuals with serious illness report a greater symptom burden than their higher-income counterparts,[79,80] yet multiple studies have found an association between low socioeconomic status (SES) and more disease-modifying care at the EOL, increased likelihood of institutional death, and a lower likelihood of receiving hospice.[81–83] Low-income hospice patients also have a decreased likelihood of remaining at home until death.[83]

As US hospice is an insurance benefit, being uninsured is a barrier to hospice. Uninsured individuals are more likely to be diagnosed at later stages of disease compared with the privately insured[84] and individuals presenting with the advanced disease tend to experience greater symptom burden, have fewer opportunities for EOL discussions, have prolonged hospitalizations, hospital death, and more ICU admissions.[85–87] Although many hospices will accept those who are uninsured or cannot self-pay, about 20% of hospices provide no charity care.[88] For-profit hospices are less likely to provide charity care than non-profit agencies.[88] As the number of for-profit hospices is growing, access to hospice among the uninsured warrants closer attention.[23,89]

NON-HOSPICE PALLIATIVE CARE

In the United States, hospital PC was developed in response to the limitations on hospice eligibility and the need to improve care for those whose serious illnesses were not yet terminal.[25,90,91] Through visionary leadership, strategic planning, and philanthropic support, PC has achieved large-scale dissemination over the past 20 years.[92] In 2001, only 7% of hospitals with 50 or more beds reported having a PC team whereas 72% of such hospitals did in 2019.[93] PC has increasingly sought to have influence in earlier stages of disease progression, to reach patients with non-cancer disease, and to become integrated into health systems.[24] Although progress toward these goals has been made, significant challenges remain.

The prognosis-based distinction between PC and hospice is unique to the United States.[90] Many seriously-ill patients who are ineligible for or who do not want hospice lack a PC alternative outside of inpatient settings resulting in significant care gaps.[94] New value-based care models including home-based PC are being developed and indicate improved patient satisfaction, improved symptom management, improved quality of life, reduced health care use, and may improve hospice utilization; however, these services are not yet widely available.[95–98] New Medicare Advantage (MA) plans have the flexibility to offer enrollees supplemental services including home-based PC, caregiver support, and transportation. These plans have the potential to customize care for seriously-ill individuals, but widespread uptake is expected to be gradual.[99]

Early research indicates geographic variation in the availability of new MA supplemental services.[100] Oversight is needed to ensure equitable care availability as these programs are increasingly being adopted.

SUMMARY

The MHB's eligibility criterion was intended to make hospice cost-neutral by ensuring that its costs would be offset by reduced expenditures for cancer-directed treatment.[101] This focus on cost containment has resulted in reduced access to hospice by many, disproportionately affecting patients with non-cancer diagnoses, minoritized individuals, and patients of lower SES. The inability to receive concurrent palliative and disease-modifying treatment forces patients to make a "terrible choice."[102] Hospice fails a test of fairness as being willing to forgo life-sustaining treatment does not identify those with a greater need for hospice services.[103]

Hospice's limited staff visits, restrictions on the use of inpatient hospice, and challenges in paying for hospice in SNFs disadvantage individuals lacking sufficient family caregivers and/or suitable housing. Hospice does not provide coverage for social support or services beyond social worker support, occasional respite care, and bereavement services. Many hospices do, however, use internal funds for social support needs not reimbursed by insurers such as food, shelter, utilities, and transportation suggesting that the current reimbursement rate inadequately addresses patients' and families' social needs.[104]

Social justice, the fair disbursement of common advantages and the sharing of common burdens, has been defined as the core value of PH. Health improvement for the population and fair treatment of the disadvantaged are two aspects of justice PH champions.[105] The development of both hospice and PC over the past 50 years has been remarkable; however, new models of PC, both hospice and non-hospice, are needed to equitably meet the expected societal burden of suffering from serious illness.

DISCLOSURE

The authors have nothing to disclose.

REFERENCES

1. Byock IR. End-of-life care: a public health crisis and an opportunity for managed care. Am J Manag Care 2001;7(12):1123–32.
2. Rao JK, Anderson LA, Smith SM. End of life is a public health issue. Am J Prev Med 2002;23(3):215–20.
3. Glasgow RE, Wagner EH, Kaplan RM, et al. If diabetes is a public health problem, why not treat it as one? A population-based approach to chronic illness. Ann Behav Med 1999;21(2):159–70.
4. National Center for Health Statistics. Deaths and Mortality. Available at: https://www.cdc.gov/nchs/fastats/deaths.htm. Published 2022. Accessed December 21, 2022.
5. Dumanovsky T, Augustin R, Rogers M, et al. The growth of palliative care in U.S. Hospitals: a status report. J Palliat Med 2016;19(1):8–15.
6. Schenker Y, Park SY, Maciasz R, et al. Do patients with advanced cancer and unmet palliative care needs have an interest in receiving palliative care services? J Palliat Med 2014;17(6):667–72.

7. Singer AE, Meeker D, Teno JM, et al. Symptom trends in the last year of life from 1998 to 2010: a cohort study. Ann Intern Med 2015;162(3):175–83.

8. Fitzsimons D, Mullan D, Wilson JS, et al. The challenge of patients' unmet palliative care needs in the final stages of chronic illness. Palliat Med 2007;21(4): 313–22.

9. Schulz R, Beach SR, Friedman EM, et al. Changing structures and processes to support family caregivers of seriously ill patients. J Palliat Med 2018;21(S2): S36–42.

10. Aldridge MD, Kelley AS. The myth regarding the high cost of end-of-life care. Am J Public Health. 2015;105(12):2411–5.

11. Chino F, Peppercorn JM, Rushing C, et al. Going for broke: a longitudinal study of patient-reported financial sacrifice in cancer care. J Oncol Pract. 2018;14(9): e533–46.

12. Yabroff KR, Lund J, Kepka D, et al. Economic burden of cancer in the United States: estimates, projections, and future research. Cancer Epidemiol Biomarkers Prev 2011;20(10):2006–14.

13. Valero-Elizondo J, Chouairi F, Khera R, et al. Atherosclerotic cardiovascular disease, cancer, and financial toxicity among adults in the United States. JACC Cardio Oncol 2021;3(2):236–46.

14. US Centers for Disease Control and Prevention. Introduction to Public Health. Available at: https://www.cdc.gov/training/publichealth101/public-health.html. Published 2021. Accessed December 20, 2022, 2021.

15. World Health Organization. Constitution. Available at: https://www.who.int/about/governance/constitution. Published 2022. Accessed January 4, 2023.

16. Obermeyer Z, Makar M, Abujaber S, et al. Association between the Medicare hospice benefit and health care utilization and costs for patients with poor-prognosis cancer. JAMA 2014;312(18):1888–96.

17. Teno JM, Shu JE, Casarett D, et al. Timing of referral to hospice and quality of care: length of stay and bereaved family members' perceptions of the timing of hospice referral. J Pain Symptom Manage. 2007;34(2):120–5.

18. Teno JM, Clarridge BR, Casey V, et al. Family perspectives on end-of-life care at the last place of care. JAMA 2004;291(1):88–93.

19. Kelley AS, Deb P, Du Q, et al. Hospice enrollment saves money for Medicare and improves care quality across a number of different lengths-of-stay. Health Aff (Millwood) 2013;32(3):552–61.

20. Wright AA, Keating NL, Balboni TA, et al. Place of death: correlations with quality of life of patients with cancer and predictors of bereaved caregivers' mental health. J Clin Oncol 2010;28(29):4457–64.

21. Bradley EH, Prigerson H, Carlson MD, et al. Depression among surviving caregivers: does length of hospice enrollment matter? Am J Psychiatry 2004; 161(12):2257–62.

22. Taylor DH Jr, Ostermann J, Van Houtven CH, et al. What length of hospice use maximizes reduction in medical expenditures near death in the US Medicare program? Soc Sci Med 2007;65(7):1466–78.

23. Medicare Payment Advisory Commission.Report to the congress: Medicare payment policy., 2022, MedPAC; Washington, DC.

24. Clark D. From margins to centre: a review of the history of palliative care in cancer. Lancet Oncol 2007;8(5):430–8.

25. Connor SR. Development of hospice and palliative care in the United States. Omega (Westport) 2007;56(1):89–99.

26. Mor V, Teno JM. Regulating and paying for hospice and palliative care: reflections on the medicare hospice benefit. J Health Polit Policy Law 2016;41(4): 697–716.
27. Greer DS, Mor V. How Medicare is altering the hospice movement. Hastings Cent Rep 1985;15(5):5–9.
28. Mor V, Greer D, Kastenbaum R. The hospice experiment. Baltimore: Johns Hopkins University Press; 1988.
29. Trandel ET, Lowers J, Bannon M, et al. Barriers to acceptance of hospice care: a randomized VIgnette-based experiment. J Gen Intern Med 2022;38(2):277–84.
30. National Hospice and Palliative Care Organization. NHPCO Facts and Figures. Alexandria, VA: NHPCO;2022. Available at: https://www.nhpco.org/wp-content/uploads/NHPCO-Facts-Figures-2020-edition.pdf.
31. Unroe KT, Greiner MA, Hernandez AF, et al. Resource use in the last 6 months of life among medicare beneficiaries with heart failure, 2000-2007. Arch Intern Med 2011;171(3):196–203.
32. Yim CK, Barron Y, Moore S, et al. Hospice enrollment in patients with advanced heart failure decreases acute medical service utilization. Circ Heart Fail 2017; 10(3):e003335.
33. Cheung WY, Schaefer K, May CW, et al. Enrollment and events of hospice patients with heart failure vs. cancer. J Pain Symptom Manage. 2013;45(3):552–60.
34. Gelfman LP, Barron Y, Moore S, et al. Predictors of hospice enrollment for patients with advanced heart failure and effects on health care use. JACC Heart Fail 2018;6(9):780–9.
35. Teno JM, Weitzen S, Fennell ML, et al. Dying trajectory in the last year of life: does cancer trajectory fit other diseases? J Palliat Med 2001;4(4):457–64.
36. Lunney JR, Lynn J, Foley DJ, et al. Patterns of functional decline at the end of life. JAMA 2003;289(18):2387–92.
37. Lunney JR, Lynn J, Hogan C. Profiles of older medicare decedents. J Am Geriatr Soc 2002;50(6):1108–12.
38. Goldstein NE, Lynn J. Trajectory of end-stage heart failure: the influence of technology and implications for policy change. Perspect Biol Med 2006;49(1):10–8.
39. Lemond L, Allen LA. Palliative care and hospice in advanced heart failure. Prog Cardiovasc Dis 2011;54(2):168–78.
40. Xu J, Nolan MT, Heinze K, et al. Symptom frequency, severity, and quality of life among persons with three disease trajectories: cancer, ALS, and CHF. Appl Nurs Res 2015;28(4):311–5.
41. Goebel JR, Doering LV, Shugarman LR, et al. Heart failure: the hidden problem of pain. J Pain Symptom Manage. 2009;38(5):698–707.
42. Yancy CW, Jessup M, Bozkurt B, et al. 2013 ACCF/AHA guideline for the management of heart failure: a report of the American college of cardiology foundation/American heart association task force on practice guidelines. J Am Coll Cardiol 2013;62(16):e147–239.
43. Gysels MH, Higginson IJ. Caring for a person in advanced illness and suffering from breathlessness at home: threats and resources. Palliat Support Care 2009; 7(2):153–62.
44. Walden JA, Dracup K, Westlake C, et al. Educational needs of patients with advanced heart failure and their caregivers. J Heart Lung Transplant 2001; 20(7):766–9.
45. Hines A.L., Barrett M.L., Jiang H.J., Steiner C.A., Conditions With the Largest Number of Adult Hospital Readmissions by Payer, 2011. In: Healthcare Cost and Utilization Project (HCUP) Statistical Briefs [Internet]. Rockville (MD):

Agency for Healthcare Research and Quality (US); 2006 Feb–. Statistical Brief #172.

46. Kheirbek RE, Fletcher RD, Bakitas MA, et al. Discharge hospice referral and lower 30-day all-cause readmission in medicare beneficiaries hospitalized for heart failure. Circ Heart Fail 2015;8(4):733–40.

47. Mitchell SL, Teno JM, Kiely DK, et al. The clinical course of advanced dementia. N Engl J Med 2009;361(16):1529–38.

48. Sachs GA, Shega JW, Cox-Hayley D. Barriers to excellent end-of-life care for patients with dementia. J Gen Intern Med 2004;19(10):1057–63.

49. Christakis NA, Escarce JJ. Survival of Medicare patients after enrollment in hospice programs. N Engl J Med 1996;335(3):172–8.

50. Walsh JS, Welch HG, Larson EB. Survival of outpatients with Alzheimer-type dementia. Ann Intern Med 1990;113(6):429–34.

51. Wolfson C, Wolfson DB, Asgharian M, et al. A reevaluation of the duration of survival after the onset of dementia. N Engl J Med 2001;344(15):1111–6.

52. Helmes E, Merskey H, Fox H, et al. Patterns of deterioration in senile dementia of the Alzheimer type. Arch Neurol 1995;52(3):306–10.

53. Volicer L. Hospice care for dementia patients. J Am Geriatr Soc 1997;45(9):1147–9.

54. Cross SH, Kaufman BG, Taylor DH Jr, et al. Trends and factors associated with place of death for individuals with dementia in the United States. J Am Geriatr Soc 2019;68(2):250–5.

55. Aragon K, Covinsky K, Miao Y, et al. Use of the Medicare posthospitalization skilled nursing benefit in the last 6 months of life. Arch Intern Med 2012;172(20):1573–9.

56. Miller SC, Teno JM, Mor V. Hospice and palliative care in nursing homes. Clin Geriatr Med 2004;20(4):717–34, vii.

57. Trivedi DD. Palliative dialysis in end-stage renal disease. Am J Hosp Palliat Care 2011;28(8):539–42.

58. Wachterman MW, Hailpern SM, Keating NL. Kurella tamura M, O'Hare AM. Association between hospice length of stay, health care utilization, and medicare costs at the end of life among patients who received maintenance hemodialysis. JAMA Intern Med 2018;178(6):792–9.

59. Miceli PJ, Mylod DE. Satisfaction of families using end-of-life care: current successes and challenges in the hospice industry. Am J Hosp Palliat Care 2003;20(5):360–70.

60. Schockett ER, Teno JM, Miller SC, et al. Late referral to hospice and bereaved family member perception of quality of end-of-life care. J Pain Symptom Manage. 2005;30(5):400–7.

61. Rickerson E, Harrold J, Kapo J, et al. Timing of hospice referral and families' perceptions of services: are earlier hospice referrals better? J Am Geriatr Soc 2005;53(5):819–23.

62. Welch LC, Teno JM, Mor V. End-of-life care in black and white: race matters for medical care of dying patients and their families. J Am Geriatr Soc 2005;53(7):1145–53.

63. Ornstein KA, Roth DL, Huang J, et al. Evaluation of racial disparities in hospice use and end-of-life treatment intensity in the REGARDS cohort. JAMA Netw Open 2020;3(8):e2014639.

64. Hanchate A, Kronman AC, Young-Xu Y, et al. Racial and ethnic differences in end-of-life costs: why do minorities cost more than whites? Arch Intern Med 2009;169(5):493–501.

65. Anderson KO, Green CR, Payne R. Racial and ethnic disparities in pain: causes and consequences of unequal care. J Pain 2009;10(12):1187–204.
66. Johnson KS, Kuchibhatla M, Tanis D, et al. Racial differences in hospice revocation to pursue aggressive care. Arch Intern Med 2008;168(2):218–24.
67. Cross SH, Warraich HJ. Changes in the place of death in the United States. N Engl J Med 2019;381(24):2369–70.
68. Smith AK, Earle CC, McCarthy EP. Racial and ethnic differences in end-of-life care in fee-for-service Medicare beneficiaries with advanced cancer. J Am Geriatr Soc 2009;57(1):153–8.
69. Lackan NA, Eschbach K, Stimpson JP, et al. Ethnic differences in in-hospital place of death among older adults in California: effects of individual and contextual characteristics and medical resource supply. Med Care. 2009;47(2): 138–45.
70. Haas JS, Earle CC, Orav JE, et al. Lower use of hospice by cancer patients who live in minority versus white areas. J Gen Intern Med 2007;22(3):396–9.
71. Cruz-Oliver DM, Sanchez-Reilly S. Barriers to quality end-of-life care for latinos: hospice health care professionals' perspective. J Hospice Palliat Nurs 2016; 18(6):505–11.
72. Selsky C, Kreling B, Luta G, et al. Hospice knowledge and intentions among Latinos using safety-net clinics. J Palliat Med 2012;15(9):984–90.
73. Kwak J, Haley WE. Current research findings on end-of-life decision making among racially or ethnically diverse groups. Gerontol 2005;45(5):634–41.
74. Ngo-Metzger Q, McCarthy EP, Burns RB, et al. Islanders dying of cancer use hospice less frequently than older white patients. Am J Med 2003;115(1):47–53.
75. Ngo-Metzger Q, Phillips RS, McCarthy EP. Ethnic disparities in hospice use among Asian-American and Pacific Islander patients dying with cancer. J Am Geriatr Soc 2008;56(1):139–44.
76. Kwak J, Salmon JR. Attitudes and preferences of Korean-American older adults and caregivers on end-of-life care. J Am Geriatr Soc 2007;55(11):1867–72.
77. Bell CL, Kuriya M, Fischberg D. Hospice referrals and code status: outcomes of inpatient palliative care consultations among Asian Americans and Pacific Islanders with cancer. J Pain Symptom Manage. 2011;42(4):557–64.
78. Enguidanos S, Yonashiro-Cho J, Cote S. Knowledge and perceptions of hospice care of Chinese older adults. J Am Geriatr Soc 2013;61(6):993–8.
79. Cimino T, Said K, Safier L, et al. Psychosocial distress among oncology patients in the safety net. Psycho Oncol 2020;29(11):1927–35.
80. Rosenzweig MQ, Althouse AD, Sabik L, et al. The association between area deprivation index and patient-reported outcomes in patients with advanced cancer. Health Equity. 2021;5(1):8–16.
81. Chang CM, Wu CC, Yin WY, et al. Low socioeconomic status is associated with more aggressive end-of-life care for working-age terminal cancer patients. Oncologist. 2014;19(12):1241–8.
82. Hardy D, Chan W, Liu CC, et al. Racial disparities in the use of hospice services according to geographic residence and socioeconomic status in an elderly cohort with nonsmall cell lung cancer. Cancer. 2011;117(7):1506–15.
83. Barclay JS, Kuchibhatla M, Tulsky JA, et al. Association of hospice patients' income and care level with place of death. JAMA Intern Med 2013;173(6):450–6.
84. Ward EM, Fedewa SA, Cokkinides V, et al. The association of insurance and stage at diagnosis among patients aged 55 to 74 years in the national cancer database. Cancer J 2010;16(6):614–21.

85. Krakauer EL, Crenner C, Fox K. Barriers to optimum end-of-life care for minority patients. J Am Geriatr Soc 2002;50(1):182–90.

86. Hui D, Kim SH, Roquemore J, et al. Impact of timing and setting of palliative care referral on quality of end-of-life care in cancer patients. Cancer. 2014;120(11):1743–9.

87. Hui D, Karuturi MS, Tanco KC, et al. Targeted agent use in cancer patients at the end of life. J Pain Symptom Manage. 2013;46(1):1–8.

88. Aldridge MD, Schlesinger M, Barry CL, et al. National hospice survey results: for-profit status, community engagement, and service. JAMA Intern Med 2014;174(4):500–6.

89. Stevenson DG, Dalton JB, Grabowski DC, et al. Nearly half of all Medicare hospice enrollees received care from agencies owned by regional or national chains. Health Aff (Millwood) 2015;34(1):30–8.

90. Meier DE. Increased access to palliative care and hospice services: opportunities to improve value in health care. Milbank Q 2011;89(3):343–80.

91. A controlled trial to improve care for seriously ill hospitalized patients. The study to understand prognoses and preferences for outcomes and risks of treatments (SUPPORT). The SUPPORT Principal Investigators. JAMA 1995;274(20):1591–8.

92. Cassel JB, Bowman B, Rogers M, et al. Palliative care leadership C. Palliative care leadership Centers are key to the diffusion of palliative care innovation. Health Aff (Millwood) 2018;37(2):231–9.

93. Center to Advance Palliative Care. America's Care of Serious Illness: A state-by-state report card on access to palliative care in our nation's hospitals. Available at: Https://Reportcard.Capc.Org/. 2019. Accessed December 20, 2022.

94. Kamal AH, Currow DC, Ritchie CS, et al. Community-based palliative care: the natural evolution for palliative care delivery in the U.S. J Pain Symptom Manage. 2013;46(2):254–64.

95. Bull J, Kamal AH, Harker M, et al. Standardization and scaling of a community-based palliative care model. J Palliat Med 2017;20(11):1237–43.

96. Lustbader D, Mudra M, Romano C, et al. The impact of a home-based palliative care program in an accountable care organization. J Palliat Med 2017;20(1):23–8.

97. Brumley R, Enguidanos S, Jamison P, et al. Increased satisfaction with care and lower costs: results of a randomized trial of in-home palliative care. J Am Geriatr Soc 2007;55(7):993–1000.

98. Taylor DH Jr, Kaufman BG, Olson A, et al. Paying for palliative care in medicare: evidence from the four seasons/duke CMMI demonstration. J Pain Symptom Manage. 2019;58(4):654–61.e2.

99. Crook H, Olson A, Alexander M, et al. Improving Serious Illness Care in Medicare Advantage: New Regulatory Flexibility for Supplemental Benefits. 2019. Available at: https://healthpolicy.duke.edu/sites/default/files/2020-07/MA_SupplementalBenefits_2019.pdf.

100. Crook HL, Zhao AT, Saunders RS. Analysis of medicare advantage plans' supplemental benefits and variation by county. JAMA Netw Open 2021;4(6):e2114359.

101. Coverage of Hospice Care Under the Medicare Program: Hearing Before the Subcommittee on Health of the Committee on Ways and Means, House of Representatives, Ninety-seventh Congress, Second Session on H.R. 5180, to Provide Hospice Care Under the Medicare Program, March 25, 1982.

102. Casarett DJ, Fishman JM, Lu HL, et al. The terrible choice: re-evaluating hospice eligibility criteria for cancer. J Clin Oncol 2009;27(6):953–9.

103. Fishman J, O'Dwyer P, Lu HL, et al. Race, treatment preferences, and hospice enrollment: eligibility criteria may exclude patients with the greatest needs for care. Cancer. 2009;115(3):689–97.

104. Boucher NA, Kuchibhatla M, Meeting Basic Needs Johnson KS, et al. By hospice. J Palliat Med 2017;20(6):642–6.

105. Powers PFR. Social justice: the moral foundations of public health and health policy. New York: Oxford University Press; 2006.

Advance Care Planning in the Geriatrics Clinic

Sivan Ben-Moshe, MD[a],*, Kimberly A. Curseen, MD, FAAHPM[b],*

KEYWORDS

- Advance care planning • Advance directives • Communication
- Current procedural terminology • Serious illness • End of life

KEY POINTS

- Advance care planning (ACP) can still serve an important role to better understand older adults' values and preferences who are diagnosed and living with a serious illness.
- ACP is reimbursable and can be incorporated into the workflow of ambulatory geriatric clinics.
- Focus of ACP should be in the conversation to determine goals and values verse completing a document. The literature on effectiveness is controversial.
- There are barriers experienced by minoritized communities, which adversely affect views and experiences with advanced care planning.

BACKGROUND

The urgency of advance care planning (ACP) came out of several monumental cases in which there were family disputes about the type of care their critically ill member would have wished for themselves.[1] Because legal battles ensued, much of the process included choosing a health-care surrogate to fulfill the wishes of the patient when there was a time the patient could no longer make decisions for themselves. This also included filling out legal forms to document those precise wishes, called advance directives.[2] Advanced directives consist of 2 parts a living-will and a medical/health-care power of attorney. A living-will is a patient facing document where the patient communicates their treatment preferences in case of serious and or catastrophic illness. In addition to treatment preferences, this document may contain wishes concerning funeral arrangements, and organ donation. A living-will can be changed based on a patient preference, which may change during the course of the illness and should

[a] Department of Medicine, Division of General Medicine and Geriatrics, Emory University School of Medicine, Geriatrics Clinic, Emory Healthcare, 1525 Clifton Road Northeast, Atlanta, GA 30322, USA; [b] Division of Palliative Medicine, Emory Palliative Care Center, 1821 Clifton Road, Northeast, Suite 1017, Atlanta, GA 30322, USA
* Corresponding authors.
E-mail addresses: sivan.ben-moshe@emory.edu (S.B.-M.); kacurseen@emory.edu (K.A.C.)

Clin Geriatr Med 39 (2023) 407–416
https://doi.org/10.1016/j.cger.2023.05.003
0749-0690/23/© 2023 Elsevier Inc. All rights reserved.

be readdressed with changes in clinical conditions.[3] A medical power of attorney allows a patient to designate a surrogate decision-maker of their choice to carry out their treatment preferences in case they are unable to meaningfully communicate their wishes. The surrogate decision-maker may be charged with making decisions in the best interest of the patient consistent with their stated values if no preferences have been previously documented or communicated. The medical power of attorney does not have to be relative of the patient.[3,4] ACP is the discussion and preparation of patients and caregivers, often guided by a health-care provider, to determine treatment preferences in case of serious illness. ACP includes but is not limited to medical preference, caregivers, living arrangements, funeral, and financial planning. ACP is a dynamic discussion that evolves at a person serious illness and needs evolve.[3–5] Both ACP and completion of advanced directives can take place in anticipation of serious illness.

However, despite all significant efforts, patients' wishes were still not being met, even till this day. The challenging work began with the 1995 landmark research trial, the SUPPORT trial "The *Study* to *Understand Prognoses* and *Preferences* for *Outcomes* and *Risks* of *Treatments* (SUPPORT)," funded by the Robert Wood Johnsen foundation in an effort to study death in America and combat the culture of denial.[6,7] Despite significant intervention in education and communication the conclusions of the SUPPORT trial again did not show significant changes in improving "end-of-life decision making and reduce the frequency of a mechanically supported, painful, and prolonged process of dying."[6] Although the trial's intervention did not yield the outcomes the designers anticipated, many in the Palliative field credit the SUPPORT trial as the catalyst for increasing the amount of evidence-based data regarding the dying process and patient preferences.[8]

Geriatrics recognizes the important of understanding patient preference, which is the primary purpose of ACP. "*What Matters Most*," which is defined by "each individual's own meaningful health outcomes goals and preferences" is the fifth M in the geriatric 5 Ms, which guides clinical care for older adults.[9]

Up until 2017, there was no general definition for the term ACP. This led to much confusion in the research space and measuring outcomes.[10,11] Many of the previous interpretations included filling out legally binding documents and code status discussions. In 2017, a group of specialists gathered to formulate a consensus definition for ACP. After much deliberation, the following was defined, "Advance care planning is a process that supports adults at any age or stage of health in understanding and sharing their personal values, life goals, and preferences regarding future medical care. The goal of advance care planning is to help ensure that people receive medical care that is consistent with their values, goals, and preferences during serious and chronic illness."[11] The definition purposefully excluded code status and filling out advance directives. This was left as a more open definition and placed emphasis on the actual conversation.

In 2016, the Centers for Medicare & Medicaid Services (CMS) decided that having these conversations was important enough that clinicians should be reimbursed for them. Therefore, 2 Current Procedural Terminology (CPT) codes for ACP took effect, 99497 and 99498.[12] As per the CMS website 99497 is "Advance care planning including the explanation and discussion of advance directives such as standard forms (with completion of such forms, when performed), by the physician or other qualified health professional; first 30 minutes, face-to-face with the patient, family member(s) and/or surrogate.[12,13] The work RVU he Centers for Medicare & Medicaid Services (CMS) recognizes two ACP codes for 99497 is 1.5 with an estimated payment of $85.99."[14] The second CPT code, 99498, is for the additional minutes of service from 46 minutes and more. This has increased the frequency of these conversations and helped incentivize clinicians willing to put in the time.[12,15]

More recently, it has been argued that discussing hypothetical scenarios is unhelpful to patients and does not achieve the desired clinical outcomes they wished for in an article by Morrison and colleagues explained, *"the assumption that ACP will result in goal-concordant end-of-life care led to widespread public initiatives promoting its use, physician reimbursement for ACP discussions, and use as a quality measure by the Centers for Medicare & Medicaid Services, commercial payers, and others. However, the scientific data do not support this assumption. ACP does not improve end-of-life care, nor does its documentation serve as a reliable and valid quality indicator of an end-of-life discussion."*[16] In a scoping review in 2020 published in the American Geriatric Society Journal suggests otherwise. When looking at more specific outcomes, it describes that ACP may be significant in the trajectory of the patient and provider relationship within the progression of a disease, although it may not always lead to patient preferences, emphasizing the conversation continues to be paramount. Further, they found numerous benefits including for the domain of Quality of care, *"88% of outcomes were positive for patient-surrogate/clinician congruence, 100% for patients/surrogate/clinician satisfaction with communication and 75% for surrogate satisfaction with patients' care, but not for goal concordance."*[17] Although it is important to note this discourse, on the micro level, the benefits of the conversation continue to outweigh the controversy, especially when it comes to the clinician–patient relationship. Numerous studies have shown it builds trust and strengthens the therapeutic bond between the 2 entities from having these conversations.[18,19] The importance of ACP is not in the document that it produces but conversation between patient and family, and patient and health-care provider concerning values.[3,5] In this case, it is important to understand why having these conversations preferably in the outpatient rather than inpatient setting is key.[17,19,20]

In the geriatric's outpatient setting, ACP can help to ensure that patients receive care that aligns with their values and preferences before arriving to the hospital and discussing preferences in highly stressful conditions. Older adults may have complex medical histories, multiple chronic conditions, and may be nearing the end of life. ACP can help to ensure that patients receive care that is consistent with their goals and values.[20]

BARRIERS TO IMPLEMENTATION

Despite the importance of ACP in the geriatric's clinic, there are several barriers to implementation. Some of the main challenges are the lack of time, staff, and training. Clinics may have limited staff and patients may not want to dedicate time in discussing their wishes, instead focus on acute issues. In addition, there may be cultural or religious barriers to ACP. Some patients may be uncomfortable discussing end-of-life issues or may have cultural beliefs that conflict with certain types of medical treatment. These barriers can make it difficult for health-care providers to initiate discussions about ACP.[21] Further, ACP can be controversial because many people are not aware of its importance or do not understand how it works. This can lead to misunderstandings, mistrust, and resistance to the process. One of the largest barriers is clinicians themselves, not initiating the topic due to their own fears about being able to communicate appropriately.[22] Another barrier is that although many countries have census for the definition of ACP not all do; for example, Indonesia does not.[23] An article in the Japanese Journal of Clinical Oncology identified several Asian countries have differing definitions of ACP and it is important to approach this topic with cultural sensitivity.[21,24]

Literature is starting to address the social determinants of health, structural and systemic racism that affects ACP and communication in minoritized groups that adversely affects the quality of ACP.[25,26] Interpersonal bias, structural racism, and economic disparities affect how patients from minoritized and vulnerable communities experience ACP. The reaction to minoritized community preferences has been to pathologize the people verse understanding reasons for treatment preference. There also is literature that shows minoritized communities that are willing to discuss ACP and goals. Minoritized communities' views on ACP and advance directives are more complex and nuanced than mistrust, spirituality, and lack of education.[27,28]

Recent data has shown even with adjusting for socioeconomic status and education, White patients were more likely to complete and be offered advanced care planning versus patients of African descent.[26] Community-based research and interventions have offered culturally sensitive approached to end-of-life discussion and ACP.[21] This has led to innovative culturally sensitive tools to facilitate advance care as well as antiracist research in this area.[28,29]

STRATEGIES FOR SUCCESSFUL IMPLEMENTATION INTO ROUTINE CLINICAL WORKFLOW

In the following sections, we will focus on who, what, when, and where health-care staff can have these conversations. According to the CMS CPT codes mentioned previously, a variety of health-care clinicians can bill for ACP services, including physicians, nurse practitioners, and physician assistants. Other health-care professionals, such as social workers and chaplains, may also be able to provide ACP services but their ability to bill for these services may depend on their scope of practice and state regulations.[15] Medicare provided no specific requirements for using ACP codes, other than it must be *voluntary* face-to-face or telemedicine discussion regarding ACP with patient, proxy, or surrogate and must be at least 16 minutes long.

Discussions can include review of relevant medical records, complex medical decision-making regarding serious illness, discussion of goals and preferences for care, explanation of relevant advance directives, including, but not requiring completion of forms.[12,15] It is important to note that reimbursement rates for ACP services may vary by insurance plan and by state, and not all insurance plans may cover ACP services.[14]

However, if a patient has enrolled in Medicare part B, they are eligible for a yearly visit called the "Annual Wellness Visit" (AWV). AWV is a preventive health-care benefit for Medicare beneficiaries in the United States. The AWV is designed to help health-care clinicians assess and improve the overall health of Medicare beneficiaries by providing personalized health advice and creating a preventive care plan. One component of the AWV is ACP discussion.[30,31] During this particular visit, when using the −33 modifier while billing for the visit, patients are not charged for an ACP conversation if you use the CPT codes stated above. Therefore, it is optimal to have these discussions during the AWV.[31] Patients also know that it is considered a "Medicare Visit" and infer that this discussion is integral to the visit and the requirements of the visit. This normalizes the discussion and allows a certain distance between the clinician and patient, considering it is standardized in the visit.

Another time to have these discussions is during posthospital visits although the data are mixed. Clinic visits may be longer for posthospital patients and allow time to review and reconcile information from the hospitalization. New information, exacerbation of chronic conditions, and changes in prognosis may arise after hospitalization, which warrant a frank discussion about future therapies and care. It is beneficial to have these discussions before any major procedure or surgery because patients may end up with serious complications that can affect their quality of life.[32]

IMPORTANT STEPS IN ACP

The first step in goals of care discussions is discussing patient's wishes. Previously, legally binding advanced directives have been used as a template to guide conversations. The issue with many of these types of forms is they may not focus on what matters most and are more concerned about types of life support therapies at the end of life.[3,16] At times, lawyers, who are not involved in medical decisions, are assisting patients in filling out these forms and the forms may be complicated in that they require a notary in some states. Therefore, new forms and new evidence-based communication aids have evolved and are being integrated into practice. A few examples are the "Five Wishes" (can be downloaded for a fee) and "Serious Illness Conversation guide (SICG)." Some of the aids such as the "Serious Illness Conversation guide" developed by Ariadne Labs, requires 2.5 to 3 hours formal training.[33,34] The basic format of the conversation is laid out in a strategic way, which allows the patient to build trust and control the conversation. Information is shared with permission from the patients and questions guide the patient in exploring their values in regard to their health. It can be performed after training by primary care and subspecialty providers. Literature has shown SICG to be feasible, acceptable and experienced positively by both patients and providers.[35] Current work is being done to adapt the guide to be more culturally sensitive.[36] Newer directives focus on a more functional based prognosis rather than a time-based prognosis. For example, one of the questions in the "Serious Illness Conversation Guide" is "If you become sicker, how much are you willing to go through for the possibility of gaining more time?"[35]

After assessing patients' health-care goals, the next step is helping patients identify a health-care proxy (HCP) that will make medical decisions on their behalf if they are unable to. At times, patients may find this process difficult. Using decision aids or other educational resources to help patients and families understand the ACP process can simplify complex medical information and may be particularly useful for patients with limited health literacy. One example is the website "prepareforyourcare.org" free of charge and also available in Spanish[19] (**Table 1**).

Once a surrogate is identified, it is important to encourage the patient to discuss their wishes with them and with any other important people in their lives. All too often, disputes originate because only the primary person knew the patient's wishes while others were left in the dark. At times, it may be too difficult for patients to discuss their wishes with others, and in these cases, it would be helpful to guide them in the discussion or offer to lead the discussion as their provider.[5,8]

The final step is documenting the HCP and the patient wishes. It is important to document the HCP because the state may appoint one for the patient if they do not have one. If a patient desires a specific person. It is in their best interest to document that person's name. For some patients, depending on their culture or family dynamics, more than one person may be the decision maker. Although the conversation is also important to document in a note or on a legally binding document, it is more important to have the conversation and make sure the patient's HCP know their wishes as well. Essential to the process is also to figure out which documents are legally binding in the patient's state of residence.[14] However, data for ACP posthospitalization for nursing home patients showed inconsistent findings. One reason posited lack of standard and clinical expertise of nursing home staff and stress importance of focus intervention designed for this population.[37] Another barrier was noted in a qualitative study

Table 1 Advance care planning tools for older patient	
INTERACT-tool; Long-term Care	https://www.med-pass.com/long-term-care/interact-version-3-0-tools/advance-care-planning-tools.html
Fair Health Consumer: Shared Decision Making	https://www.fairhealthconsumer.org/shared-decision-making
PREPARE for your care	https://prepareforyourcare.org/en/welcome (video)
The Conversation Project	https://theconversationproject.org/nhdd/advance-care-planning/
Respecting Choices	https://respectingchoices.org/
Loving Conversations	http://www.healthlawyers.org
The African American Spiritual and Ethical Guide to End of Life Care – What Y'all Gon' Do with Me?	https://eolcareguide.org/
Five Wishes	https://www.fivewishes.org/for-myself/
End of Life Decision: Honoring the Wishes of the Person with Alzheimer's Disease	http://www.alz.org/national/documents/brochure_endoflifedecisions.pdf
Consumer's Tool Kit for Health Care Advance Planning	https://apps.americanbar.org/aging/publications/docs/consumer

Common validated tools used for advanced care planning tool on line for provider and patient reference.
Refs.[21,34]

that some patients found the discussion more difficult and to be in sharp contrast to the focus in the hospital, which was to clinically improve. However, some patients found it motivating to discuss ACP for their and their families future.[38]

Most states have a specific advance directive form and also a variation of a Medical/ Physician Orders for Life-Sustaining Treatment (MOLST/POLST), which is medical document. POLST/MOLST does not replace an advanced directive; it can serve as a complement. POLST is document of medical orders that is appropriate to complete if the patient if medically fragility, and has serious illness nearing the end of life. This document is completed with a health-care provider and patient/surrogate. It is intended to be a portable document that can be taken to different levels of care to make sure patients end of life preferences are honored. This document clarifies code status, preferences for hospitalization, life support, antibiotics, and artificial nutrition and hydration. It also requires yearly review.[39] Not all states or health-care entities recognized these as actionable medical orders. The concern may be inability to validate the medical privileges or competency of the completing provider, and inability to verify circumstances or conditions under which the document was completed. If that is the case, the document serves as only as a complement to advance directives.

As stated previously, these forms may not focus on what matters most and are more concerned about types of life support therapies at the end of life. Therefore, an additional note in the patient's medical record including the contents of the discussion would be helpful.[40,41]

For patients with dementia and ACP, it is always best to try to have these conversations earlier in the course of the disease, so they can be full present in understanding their choices. However, even in later stages of the disease, if they continue to be verbal, and may still have some capacity to make decisions, it is important to try to have conversations because they may be able to share specific information regarding their health-care wishes. Sometimes, they can at least identify an HCP they trust.[42,43] They may also understand questions involving values more than those loaded with medical jargon. Therefore, it is recommended to gauge their level of understanding and consider having a simplified discussion with them.[43]

SUMMARY

Much has been said about ACP in the last 30 years, and despite the pessimistic view of some, progress has been made in the fields of communication training, proper re-imbursements, and most importantly in the culture surrounding the dying process. As it stands, the American health-care system is fragmented, expensive, and discrimina-tory. There are countless variables in the patient–clinician–surrogate dyad to draw conclusions for any one specific patient. Each individual patient, considering their cul-ture, life experiences and health-care needs should have a conversation that may one day lead to their desired health outcome. Research may not always be able to mea-sure the true impact of these conversations on the micro level and to dismiss the whole process without a reasonable alternative, considering the current challenges in the health-care system, would be a disservice to our patients, their caregivers, and their clinicians. Focusing on increasing resources in the outpatient setting to allow patients the time and space to process their challenges, desires, and needs is key to obtain successful outcomes and measures.

CLINICS CARE POINTS

- There is still place for advance care planning for geriatric patients per medical evidence.
- Advance care planning discussions should be approached with cultural humility and tailored to patient's cultural and personal values.
- Advance care planning should start in the outpatient setting and the discussion should evolve overtime as a patient clinical condition changes.
- Advance care planning is not just limited end of life and code status discussion. It should also address goals for living, financial planning, long-term dispostion and care needs.
- Provider will need to education themselves on advanced care planning reimburstment to make this this practice sustainable in geriatric and primary care clinic that service older adults.

DISCLOSURE

The authors have no relevant disclosure.

REFERENCES

1. Struck BD, Brown EA, Madison S. Advance care planning in the outpatient geri-atric medicine setting. Prim Care Clin Off Pract 2017;44(3):511–8.
2. Luce JM. A history of resolving conflicts over end-of-life care in intensive care units in the United States. Crit Care Med 2010;38(8):1623–9.
3. Auriemma CL, O'Donnell H, Klaiman T, et al. How traditional advance directives undermine advance care planning: if you have it in writing, you do not have to worry about it. JAMA Intern Med 2022;182(6):682–4.

4. Myers J, Cosby R, Gzik D, et al. Provider tools for advance care planning and goals of care discussions: a systematic review. Am J Hosp Palliat Med 2018; 35(8):1123–32.

5. Song M-K, Ward SE, Fine JP, et al. Advance care planning and end-of-life decision making in dialysis: a randomized controlled trial targeting patients and their surrogates. Am J Kidney Dis 2015;66(5):813–22.

6. Knaus W, Lynn J. Study to Understand Prognoses and Preferences for Outcomes and Risks of Treatment (SUPPORT) and Hospitalized Elderly Longitudinal Project (HELP), 1989-1997. Inter-university Consortium for Political and Social Research (distributor); 2020.

7. Kaufman SR. Intensive care, old age, and the problem of death in America. Gerontol 1998;38(6):715–25.

8. Teno JM. Lessons learned and not learned from the SUPPORT project13. Thousand Oaks, CA: Sage Publications Sage CA; 1999. p. 91–3.

9. Monette PJ, Schwartz AW. Optimizing Medications with the geriatrics 5Ms: an age-Friendly approach. Drugs Aging 2023;1–6.

10. Knight K. 50 Years of advance care planning: what do we call success? Monash Bioeth Rev 2021;39(1):28–50.

11. Sudore RL, Lum HD, You JJ, et al. Defining advance care planning for adults: a consensus definition from a multidisciplinary Delphi panel. J Pain Symptom Manag 2017;53(5):821–32. e821.

12. Belanger E, Loomer L, Teno JM, et al. Early utilization patterns of the new Medicare procedure codes for advance care planning. JAMA Intern Med 2019;179(6): 829–30.

13. Ladin K, Bronzi OC, Gazarian PK, et al. Understanding the Use of Medicare procedure codes for advance care planning: a National qualitative study: study examines the use of Medicare procedure codes for advance care planning. Health Aff 2022;41(1):112–9.

14. Dixon J, Matosevic T, Knapp M. The economic evidence for advance care planning: systematic review of evidence. Palliative medicine 2015;29(10):869–84.

15. Jones CA, Acevedo J, Bull J, et al. Top 10 tips for using advance care planning codes in palliative medicine and beyond. J Palliat Med 2016;19(12):1249–53.

16. Morrison RS, Meier DE, Arnold RM. What's wrong with advance care planning? JAMA 2021;326(16):1575–6.

17. McMahan RD, Tellez I, Sudore RL. Deconstructing the complexities of advance care planning outcomes: what do we know and where do we go? A scoping review. J Am Geriatr Soc 2021;69(1):234–44.

18. Lum HD, Dukes J, Daddato AE, et al. Effectiveness of advance care planning group visits among older adults in primary care. J Am Geriatr Soc 2020;68(10): 2382–9.

19. Freytag J, Street RL Jr, Barnes DE, et al. Empowering older adults to discuss advance care planning during clinical visits: the PREPARE randomized trial. J Am Geriatr Soc 2020;68(6):1210–7.

20. Berntsen GKR, Dalbakk M, Hurley J, et al. Person-centred, integrated and proactive care for multi-morbid elderly with advanced care needs: a propensity score-matched controlled trial. BMC Health Serv Res 2019;19(1):1–17.

21. Cain CL, Surbone A, Elk R, et al. Culture and palliative care: preferences, communication, meaning, and mutual decision making. J Pain Symptom Manag 2018;55(5):1408–19.

22. Jimenez G, Tan WS, Virk AK, et al. State of advance care planning research: a descriptive overview of systematic reviews. Palliat Support Care 2019;17(2):234–44.
23. Putranto R, Mudjaddid E, Shatri H, et al. Development and challenges of palliative care in Indonesia: role of psychosomatic medicine. Biopsychosoc Med 2017;11:1–5.
24. Cheng S-Y, Lin C-P, Chan HY-I, et al. Advance care planning in Asian culture. Jpn J Clin Oncol 2020;50(9):976–89.
25. Jones T, Luth EA, Lin S-Y, et al. Advance care planning, palliative care, and end-of-life care interventions for racial and ethnic underrepresented groups: a systematic review. J Pain Symptom Manag 2021;62(3):e248–60.
26. McDonnell J. Unraveling the effects of social class and systemic racism on advance care planning. Innovation in Aging 2020;4(Suppl 1):472.
27. Sanders JJ, Johnson KS, Cannady K, et al. From barriers to assets: rethinking factors impacting advance care planning for African Americans. Palliat Support Care 2019;17(3):306–13.
28. Johnson KS, Kuchibhatla M, Tulsky JA. What explains racial differences in the use of advance directives and attitudes toward hospice care? J Am Geriatr Soc 2008;56(10):1953–8.
29. Ejem DB, Barrett N, Rhodes RL, et al. Reducing disparities in the quality of palliative care for older African Americans through improved advance care planning: study design and protocol. J Palliat Med 2019;22(S1). S-90-S-100.
30. Nothelle SK, McGuire M, Boyd CM, et al. Effects of screening for geriatric conditions and advance care planning at the Medicare Annual Wellness Visit. J Am Geriatr Soc 2022;70(2):579–84.
31. Colburn JL, Nothelle S. The Medicare annual wellness visit. Clin Geriatr Med 2018;34(1):1–10.
32. Shah SK, Manful A, Reich AJ, et al. Advance care planning among Medicare beneficiaries with dementia undergoing surgery. J Am Geriatr Soc 2021;69(8):2273–81.
33. Daubman B-R, Bernacki R, Stoltenberg M, et al. Best practices for teaching clinicians to use a serious illness conversation guide. Palliative Medicine Reports 2020;1(1):135–42.
34. Atherton KN. Project Five Wishes: promoting advance directives in primary care. Journal of the American Association of Nurse Practitioners 2020;32(10):689–95.
35. Paladino J, Koritsanszky L, Nisotel L, et al. Patient and clinician experience of a serious illness conversation guide in oncology: a descriptive analysis. Cancer Med 2020;9(13):4550–60.
36. Beddard-Huber E, Gaspard G, Yue K. Adaptations to the serious illness conversation guide to be more culturally safe. International Journal of Indigenous Health 2021;16(1).
37. Happ MB, Capezuti E, Strumpf NE, et al. Advance care planning and end-of-life care for hospitalized nursing home residents. J Am Geriatr Soc 2002;50(5):829–35.
38. Peck V, Valiani S, Tanuseputro P, et al. Advance care planning after hospital discharge: qualitative analysis of facilitators and barriers from patient interviews. BMC Palliat Care 2018;17:1–11.
39. Mack DS, Dosa D. Improving advanced care planning through physician orders for life-sustaining treatment (POLST) expansion across the United States: lessons learned from state-based developments. Am J Hosp Palliat Med 2020;37(1):19–26.

40. Vranas KC, Plinke W, Bourne D, et al. The influence of POLST on treatment inten-sity at the end of life: a systematic review. J Am Geriatr Soc 2021;69(12):3661–74.
41. Tetrault A, Nyback M-H, Vaartio-Rajalin H, et al. Advance care planning in demen-tia care: Wants, beliefs, and insight. Nurs Ethics 2022;29(3):696–708.
42. Dening KH, Jones L, Sampson EL. Advance care planning for people with de-mentia: a review. Int Psychogeriatr 2011;23(10):1535–51.
43. Harrison Dening K, Sampson EL, De Vries K. Advance care planning in dementia: recommendations for healthcare professionals. Palliat Care Res Treat 2019;12. 1178224219826579.

Caring for Veterans with Serious Illness

Lawson J. Marcewicz, MD[a,b,*], Lynn B. O'Neill, MD[a,b],
Lauren E. Sigler, MD[a,b]

KEYWORDS

- Veterans • Serious illness • Military culture • Mental health
- Veterans Health Administration

KEY POINTS

- US Veterans comprise approximately 7% of the population. About half of these Veterans seek care within the Department of Veterans Affairs; the other half receive their health-care services in the wider community.
- The Veteran population is aging, with about half of Veterans aged older than 65 years.
- Community providers should be familiar with the unique needs of Veterans and the resources that exist to provide optimal care.

INTRODUCTION

Veterans, citizens who have served in the Uniformed Services of the United States (Army, Navy, Air Force, Marines, and Commissioned Corps of both the Public Health Service and the National Oceanic and Atmospheric Association), are an important sector of the population. An estimated 6.4% of Americans identify as Veterans[1] but this percentage is not evenly distributed among age groups. About 50% of Veterans are aged older than 65 years, with about 25% being in the 65 to 74 years age group and 25% aged 75 years or older.[1] According to US Census data, the number of individuals identifying as Veterans has declined steadily during the course of the last 2 decades.[2] During the past 20 years, the percentage of Veterans from the Korean and World War II eras has declined as these Veterans approach end-of-life, whereas the proportion of Veterans who served during the Vietnam era—about a third—has remained steady. Veterans are overwhelmingly white and men.[2]

[a] Department of Veterans Affairs, Atlanta Veterans Affairs Health Care System, 1670 Clairmont Road, Decatur, GA 30033, USA; [b] Division of Palliative Medicine, Department of Family and Preventive Medicine, Emory University School of Medicine, 1821 Clifton Road Northeast, Atlanta, GA 30329, USA
* Corresponding author.
E-mail address: lawson.marcewicz@emory.edu

Clin Geriatr Med 39 (2023) 417–422
https://doi.org/10.1016/j.cger.2023.05.001
0749-0690/23/Published by Elsevier Inc.
geriatric.theclinics.com

Literature about caring for aging Veterans and Veterans with life-limiting illness focuses in large part on conditions given special attention by the Departments of Veterans Affairs (VA) and Defense. Trainings within the VA about Veteran populations, for instance, focus on posttraumatic stress disorder (PTSD), military sexual trauma, and traumatic brain injury, as well as exposures particular to certain military conflicts, such as Agent Orange in Vietnam or burn pits in Southwest Asia.[3,4]

In this review of caring for Veterans at end-of-life, we think it is important to focus on culture as well as conditions, and that having an appreciation for and baseline understanding of Veteran culture is imperative to caring for them well. Uniformed service is a unique undertaking that carries with it experiences not easily replicated in other settings.[3,4] These experiences, some profound and some mundane, inform the creation of a culture that influences health behaviors. As with other cultures based on ethnicity, religion, or social identity, using lenses of cultural competence and humility are best practices that can assist clinicians in providing high-quality patient-centered care.

Cultural *competence* was a term first used in the health-care setting in 1989 by Cross and colleagues[5] and was specifically in reference to institutions rather than individuals. In her monograph, Cross described 5 attributes of a culturally competent organization, including "cultural self-assessment," and "consciousness of the dynamics of cultural interaction."[5] Cultural *humility* is a term that has come into vogue more recently that aims to focus more on self-awareness of providers rather than cultural knowledge or familiarity and acknowledges the complexity of overlapping cultures. In practice, cultural competence can involve growing in knowledge about other cultures and about the cultural biases that undergird an institution's practices; cultural humility in many ways supplements this, and advocates adding to cultural knowledge an awareness that a culture is neither monomorphic nor the sole influence on an individual's identity and aims to move providers away from assuming that they know or understand everything about an individual because of cultural familiarity.[5,6]

In this review, we give an overview of 3 important aspects of Veteran culture and how these aspects may influence health behaviors at end-of-life and when facing serious illness. We also discuss conditions that disproportionately affect Veterans, and how these conditions influence end-of-life care for Veterans.

VETERAN CULTURE

Veteran culture is in large part informed by and based on military culture, given that Veterans are defined as such by their military service. Unique features of military culture include its social cohesion and hierarchical organization, which are related to each other.[7] These aspects, in turn, have implications for Veteran engagement with the health-care system.

Social and task cohesion are hallmarks of military culture and have been written about in cross-cultural military contexts.[3,8,9] Cohesion is necessary to the overall function of the military—whether a military group is fighting a conflict, conducting humanitarian or natural disaster relief operations, engaging in search and rescue, or filling any of its additional roles, individuals must efficiently and effectively sublimate personal interests—such as being with family—to social or group goals. Cohesion in military units can be influenced by personal bonds between individuals but is often also *task* cohesion, "shared commitment …to achieving a goal that requires the collective efforts of the group."[9] Cohesion is created by socialization rituals, such as basic training, initiation rituals and ceremonies, and the sharing of myths.[5,8,10]

An important adjunct to building cohesiveness is hierarchical organization of military units at all levels. This hierarchical organization defines clear roles and responsibilities for all players and defines the constraints under which the organization operates. Military hierarchy allows for the accountability and order necessary to conduct operations, such as war, that place its members under extreme stress and ask them to execute acts, such as killing, that are taboo under normal social circumstances. Hierarchy functions through a modicum of extreme control over not only the actions of individuals but, at times, also their emotions: military members "master the external situation in which they find themselves through a process of gaining control over their own emotions."[5] The "warrior ethos" often stresses the importance of stoicism, self-sufficiency, and strength in this process.

These cultural perspectives and values may influence health behaviors. Mental health providers have long recognized, for instance, that ingrained stoicism and emotional control can lead to stigma around help-seeking.[11,12] In Veterans dealing with serious or life-limiting illness, this may manifest as reticence to acknowledge a decrease in independence, desire to avoid being a burden to family and loved ones, and at times minimizing the severity of pain and other symptoms. Respect for and familiarity with a hierarchy can mean that some Veterans expect—and even desire—a paternalistic approach from their health-care providers.[10] Although shared decision-making remains important when working with Veterans, they may defer to health-care teams for their expertise and recommendations before making decisions and may appreciate more direct communication about medical care.

It is important to recognize that Veteran culture does not exist in isolation. Individual experiences and interactions within the health-care system are not defined solely by Veteran culture but also by the intersectionality of such components as race, ethnicity, religious, and gender identities. Veteran culture should not be understood in a narrow purview confining Veterans to a unidimensional experience but rather as one piece of a comprehensive cultural identity.

VETERAN CONDITIONS

Some conditions are more common in Veterans than in the general population, and these conditions may have important ramifications for providers caring for Veterans.

Cancer is more common in Veterans, owing to a variety of exposures in service.[13–15] Many cancers, such as prostate cancer, lymphoma, myeloma, and amyloidosis, are linked to exposure to Agent Orange, an herbicide famously used during the Vietnam War. Other cancers may be linked either to exposures in military occupations to solvents, radiation, pesticides, and lead or to toxic exposures from the environment. Leukemia, as well as liver, bladder, and kidney cancers, have all been linked to water contamination from Camp Lejeune, for instance; many Veterans of the wars in Southwest Asia (including operations in Iraq and Afghanistan) have been exposed to burn pits, and although linkages to cancers have not been established at this time, there is a registry for these Veterans for potential health effects to be tracked.

Importantly, some Veterans with cancer may be eligible for service connection, a level of monetary compensation for Veterans whose illnesses are linked to their service in the military. Other service-connected conditions aside from cancer include amyotrophic lateral sclerosis, some forms of hepatitis and liver disease, and head and neck cancers, all of which may make Veterans eligible for service-connected compensation.

Additional comorbidities in Veterans include mental health conditions such as PTSD and substance use. A number of these conditions are more prevalent in Veterans compared with the general population and can be associated with increased symptom burden in the context of serious illness and at end-of-life.[15,16] Mental health conditions are frequently underrecognized and underdiagnosed and often manifest over time, even years following active service. PTSD develops after witnessing events perceived to be a threat to one's existence, which may include combat or seeing dead bodies. It is characterized by intrusive thoughts, avoidance of triggering events or experiences, and hypervigilance, which may manifest as irritability, insomnia, and hypervigilance. Estimated prevalence of PTSD in Veterans varies widely (anywhere from 11% to 79%)[16] and may depend on branch of military service, era, and combat exposure. Other mental health issues that affect Veterans include suicide, which occurs in Veterans at a rate about 1.5 times higher than the general population, substance use disorders, and moral injury.[16,17] Many of these conditions coexist.

Moral injury describes a distressing experience that conflicts with one's moral beliefs and values, often resulting in significant social, spiritual, and existential distress.[17] There is no consensus of what defines moral injury, although it is often marked by feelings of alienation, regret, and shame. Potentially morally injurious events may include betrayal from authority figures or other service members as well as perpetrating or witnessing others enact transgressions, such as killing in combat or failing to perform a duty. Incidence of moral injury is reported to be as high as 42% in combat Veterans regardless of service era.[17] Repeated moral injury may result in cumulative stress and an increased risk of poor health outcomes.

Traumatic experiences and mental health conditions may influence health behaviors in a number of ways. Trauma-informed care considers how common treatment modalities may trigger patients to reexperience trauma and worsen symptoms and instead seeks to focus on individual Veteran considerations and treatment approaches.[18,19]

THE VETERANS HEALTH ADMINISTRATION

The Department of VA is an executive-level cabinet within the federal government responsible for overseeing benefits for Veterans. These benefits are diverse and include items such as VA home loans and the GI Bill, among others. The VA is divided into the Veterans Benefits Administration and the Veterans Health Administration (VHA). This latter organization provides government-subsidized health care to Veterans who have served a specified amount of time on active duty. The VHA is the largest integrated health-care system in the United States and serves approximately 9 million Veterans. Despite the size and availability of health care through the VHA, about half of the country's Veterans receive their care outside of the VHA, in the community. Community providers should, therefore, be familiar with VA-based care and benefits, which can be significantly helpful for Veterans with serious illness or approaching end-of-life.[14,15]

Some of these benefits are VHA-based programs. These include Aid and Attendance, the Caregiver Support Program, and Home-Based Primary Care. Aid and Attendance and the Caregiver Support Program can provide resources—including financial support—to eligible Veterans and their families to assist with caregiving. Home-Based Primary Care delivers primary care services to Veterans in their home. To receive any of these services, Veterans must meet the program requirements, which may include serving during certain eras or having certain diseases or needs and must be enrolled within the VHA system.

Another important benefit is the availability of hospice services for Veterans. The VHA is committed to providing hospice services for Veterans who qualify. Funding is available for Veterans who do not have another payment source or otherwise need to use VHA funds for hospice care. Since 2018, the VHA has worked to increase engagement with community hospice partners and ensure that Veterans have reliable access to hospice and palliative care. The "We Honor Veterans" initiative, a partnership between community hospices and the VA to improve familiarity with Veteran-specific needs, considerations, and benefits, is an example of this.[20] The VA also makes concurrent care available for Veterans; through the VA, Veterans can receive both hospice care and disease-directed care with palliative intent when their prognoses are less than 6 months.

SUMMARY

Veterans comprise a unique subset of the population with distinctive medical and psychosocial needs. Military culture often pervades Veteran perception of and engagement in health care. Many Veterans receive medical care outside of the VHA, and it is essential for community clinicians to have a familiarity with Veteran culture, conditions, and resources available to effectively support Veterans with serious illness and at end-of-life.

CLINICS CARE POINTS

- Emphasis on social cohesion, hierarchy, and the "warrior ethos" are embedded in Veteran culture and often influence Veteran health behaviors.
- Veterans are at increased risk for cancers owing to service-related exposures as well as mental health conditions that may manifest years following active duty.
- VA-based resources available for seriously ill Veterans include financial support, home-based care, caregiving assistance, and concurrent hospice care for those who qualify.

DISCLOSURE

The authors have nothing to disclose.

REFERENCES

1. Gilligan, C. Who are America's Veterans?. In: US News and World Report. Available at: https://www.usnews.com/news/best-states/articles/2022-11-11/who-are-americas-veterans. Accessed December 16 , 2022.
2. Who are our nation's Veterans and how is their standard of living changing? In: USA Facts. Available at: https://usafacts.org/articles/who-are-our-nations-veterans-and-how-is-their-standard-of-living-changing/. Accessed December 16, 2022.
3. Richard-Eaglin A, Campbell JG, Utley-Smith Q. The aging veteran population: promoting awareness to influence best practices. Geriatr Nurs 2020;41:505–7.
4. Strom TQ, Gavian ME, Possis E, et al. Cultural and ethical considerations when working with military personnel and veterans: a primer for VA training programs. Train Educ Prof Psychol 2012;6(2):67–75.
5. Cross TL, Bazron BJ, Dennis KW, et al. Towards a culturally competent system of care. CASSP Technical Assistance Center. Washington, DC: Georgetown University Child Development Center; 1989.
6. Tervalon M, Murray-Garcia J. Cultural humility versus cultural competence: a critical distinction in defining physician training outcomes in multicultural education. J Health Care Poor Underserved 1998;9:117–25.
7. Hobbs K. Reflections on the culture of veterans. AAOHN J 2008;56(8):337–41.

8. Braswell H, Kushner HI. Suicide, social integration and masculinity in the U.S. military. Soc Sci Med 2012;74:530–6.
9. MacCoun RJ, Kier E, Belkin A. Does social cohesion determine motivation in combat: an old question with an old answer. Armed Forces Soc 2006;32(4):646–54.
10. Halden P, Jackson P. Transforming warriors: the ritual organization of military force. New York: Routledge; 2016.
11. Reger MA, Etherage JR, Reger GM, et al. Civilian psychologists in an army culture: the ethical challenge of cultural competence. Mil Psychol 2008;20:21–35.
12. Weiss E, Coll JE. The influence of military culture and veteran worldviews on mental health treatment: practice implications for combat veteran help-seeking and wellness. Int J Health, Wellness Soc 2011;1(2):75–86.
13. Thomas ML. Veterans with cancer: providing care in the community. Clin J Oncol Nurs 2020;24(3):331–5.
14. Rivera ML, Coplan B. Caring for veterans in the private sector. J Am Acad Physician Assist 2015;28(11):23–7.
15. Way D, Ersek M, Montagnini M, et al. Top ten tips palliative care providers should know about caring for veterans. Palliat Med 2019;22(6):708–13.
16. King PR, Wray LO. Managing behavioral health needs of Veterans with traumatic brain injury (TBI) in primary care. J Clin Psychol Med Settings 2012;19:376–92.
17. Norman SB, Nichter B, Maguen S, et al. Moral injury among U.S. combat Veterans with and without PTSD and depression. J Psychiatr Res 2022;154:190–7.
18. Tanielian T, Jaycox LH, Schell TL, et al. Invisible wounds: mental health and cognitive care needs of America's returning veterans. Santa Monica (CA): Rand Corporation; 2008. Available at: https://www.rand.org/pubs/research_briefs/RB9336.html.
19. Kelly U, Boyd MA, Valente SM, et al. Trauma-informed care: keeping mental health settings safe for Veterans. Issues Ment Health Nurs 2014;35. 413-319.
20. We Honor Veterans. Available at: https://www.wehonorveterans.org. Accessed December 11, 2022.

Psychedelics and Related Pharmacotherapies as Integrative Medicine for Older Adults in Palliative Care

Kabir Nigam, MD, MRes[a,b,*], Kimberly A. Curseen, MD, FAAHPM[c], Yvan Beaussant, MD, MSc[b,d]

KEYWORDS

- Existential distress • Serious illness • Palliative care • End of life • Psychedelics
- Integrative medicine • Psychedelic-assisted therapy • PAT

KEY POINTS

- Psychological distress in elderly patients undergoing palliative care is a multidimensional interplay including psychosocial and existential distress as well as physical symptom burden.
- Currently available pharmacotherapies for psychological distress in palliative care are limited and show mixed efficacy.
- Psychedelic-assisted therapy may help address existential distress by using the nonordinary state of consciousness induced to facilitate the process of meaning-making.
- Ketamine and cannabis may safely provide quick and effective symptom relief from both a physical and psychological standpoint, although more data is needed.

INTRODUCTION

With medical advancements promoting increased longevity, the number of older adults in the population is rapidly growing. Correspondingly, the prevalence of older adults affected by serious illness is increasing, and as such, the need for palliative care services is growing.[1] Patients with serious illness receiving palliative care experience numerous benefits, including improved quality of life and survival, decreased anxiety and depressive symptoms, reduced rates of hospitalization, and higher overall satisfaction.[2] Despite this, palliative care services remain underutilized. Initiation of palliative services often begins in the inpatient setting, and outpatient access to

[a] Department of Psychiatry, Brigham and Women's Hospital, 60 Fenwood Road, Boston, MA 02115, USA; [b] Harvard Medical School; [c] Division of Palliative Care, Emory University, 1821 Clifton Road, NE, Suite 1017, Atlanta, GA 30329, USA; [d] Department of Psychosocial Oncology and Palliative Care, Dana Farber Cancer Institute, 375 Longwood Avenue, Boston, MA 02115, USA
* Corresponding author.
E-mail address: knigam@partners.org

Clin Geriatr Med 39 (2023) 423–436
https://doi.org/10.1016/j.cger.2023.04.004
0749-0690/23/© 2023 Elsevier Inc. All rights reserved.
geriatric.theclinics.com

palliative services before hospitalization is limited, despite evidence supporting the integration of palliative services early in illness trajectory.[3] Furthermore, epidemiological data shows that the probability of receiving palliative care decreases with increased age despite a high need for palliative services in this population.[4]

Among the myriad of symptoms experienced by patients with serious illness, psychological distress occurs 2 to 3 times more frequently in this population than in the general population, with up to 1 in 3 patients with cancer meeting diagnostic and statistical manual (DSM) criteria for a psychiatric illness within the initial 5 years of diagnosis.[5] Patients with serious illness experiencing psychological distress are more likely to express a desire for hastened death. Additionally, patients' family members are more likely to experience an extended and more complicated grief and bereavement process.[6,7] Although currently available pharmacologic interventions may address symptom burden caused by psychological distress at the end of life, data surrounding the available pharmacotherapies has shown mixed efficacy.[8,9]

Although patients with serious illness may meet DSM criteria for various psychiatric diagnoses, the phenomenology of psychological distress in this population is unique as compared with the general population. Complicating the nuanced nature of psychological distress in palliative patients is the interplay between physical symptom burden and psychological distress, with high symptom burden being associated with greater psychological distress.[10] Although symptoms such as hopelessness, depression, and anxiety are common, these symptoms often originate from more nuanced feelings of demoralization, mourning losses (functionality, relationships, and so forth), shifting identities, death anxiety, and others, notably all in the setting of the threat of the loss of life.[5] This process is compounded in geriatric patients, where functional and interpersonal losses occur as a natural result of aging.[11] As such, the constructs of demoralization syndrome and/or death anxiety are increasingly used within palliative care to diagnose existential distress in addition to or independently of DSM diagnoses such as depression or anxiety.[12]

In this article, we will discuss the use of emerging pharmacotherapies that may help address the multidimensional nature of psychological distress in older adults in palliative care. With the increase of research into psychedelic-assisted therapy (PAT) for various psychiatric disorders, we will review the data investigating the use of PAT as a novel treatment of psychological and existential distress in palliative care. We will also discuss the evidence surrounding ketamine as an intervention for the alleviation of psychiatric symptoms. Finally, we will discuss the role of cannabis in palliative care, focusing on data related to its effect on quality of life and symptom burden.

DISCUSSION
Psychedelic-Assisted Therapy

PAT is a reemerging intervention that focuses on using psychedelic medicines to create a transient change in consciousness with the goal of facilitating and accelerating psychotherapy. The process occurs in 3 phases: preparation, dosing, and integration (Fig. 1). The majority of research using PAT within palliative care has utilized "classical" psychedelics. This term is used to describe any medicine that has intrinsic agonist/partial agonist activity at the serotonin 2A receptor, which is the primary receptor responsible for facilitating the psychedelic experience for classical psychedelics. Within the context of treating psychological distress in palliative care, research has utilized psilocybin, lysergic acid diethylamide (LSD), and dipropyltryptamine (DPT).[13] "Nonclassical" psychedelics involve mechanisms other than agonist/partial agonist activity at the serotonin 2A receptor (further discussed below), and

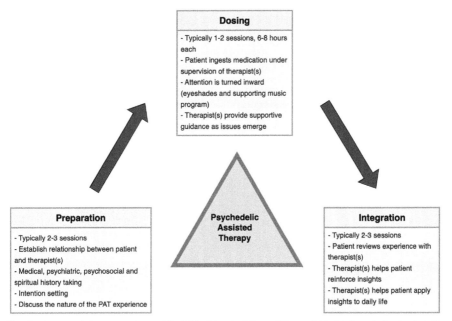

Fig. 1. Accepted framework used in PAT. *Adapted from* Ethun, C.G., Mehmet, B., Jani, A.B., et al. (2017). Frailty and cancer: implications for oncology surgery, medical oncology, and radiation oncology. A Cancer Journal for Clinicians, 67(1), 363-377.

within the context of treating psychological distress in palliative care, research has used 3,4-methylenedioxymethamphetamine (MDMA) and ketamine (**Table 1**).

Lysergic acid diethylamide and dipropyltryptamine
Before 2000, a majority of the research utilizing psychedelics used LSD due to the introduction of the compound in 1947 by Sandoz Laboratories as a psychiatric treatment, making it legally available for use in research. Regarding specifically life-threatening illness, some of the first studies using LSD were done in this population. In 1964, Kast and colleagues published a study looking at the analgesic effects of LSD in patients with terminal cancer, finding not only superior efficacy compared with hydromorphone regarding pain control but also observed changes in attitudes toward death and dying in study participants. Kast and colleagues went on to further investigate the use of LSD in end-of-life anxiety within the palliative population throughout the 1960s, treating a total of 247 terminal cancer patients with LSD.[14]

Building on this data, a group of investigators at Spring Grove State Hospital conducted a series of studies between the late 1960s and mid-1970s aimed at using LSD to facilitate a "psychological peak experience" in patients with end-of-life anxiety. The protocol they created has become the foundation for modern psychedelic therapy consisting of preparation, dosing, and integration. During the course of these years, the group treated around 53 cancer patients with LSD (200–500 μg). In one trial of 22 patients, 14 showed clinically meaningful improvement, with 6 showing what was described as dramatic improvement. In another trial of 31 patients, 22 patients showed clinically meaningful improvement, with 9 showing dramatic improvement. Interestingly, for both studies, they found a correlation between the degree of improvement and the degree of the mystical experience induced by PAT, describing

Table 1
Classical and nonclassical psychedelics used in clinical trials in patients with serious illness

Classical Psychedelics (naturally occurring or synthesized from natural compounds)

Psilocybin	• Naturally occurring Schedule 1 tryptamine and 5-HT$_{2A}$ receptor agonist found in many species of mushroom, used widely as sacrament for spiritual healing, most notably among the Mazatec peoples of Oaxaca, Mexico[a] • Clinical and research use is favored due to the relatively short duration of action (4–6 h) and favorable safety profile with FDA Breakthrough Therapy designation in 2018 • Currently in phase 2 clinical trials for various mental health indications including major-depressive disorder, treatment-resistant depression, generalized anxiety disorder, and tobacco and alcohol-use disorders • Palliative care indications currently in phase 2 study include cancer-related anxiety, depression, and demoralization at end of life as well as depressive symptoms in COVID-frontline health-care workers
LSD-25	• Schedule 1 chemical derivative from ergot alkaloid in 1938 but psychoactive properties were not discovered until 1943 ushering in the first wave of public and psychiatric interest and experimentation in psychedelics in the 1950s and 1960s • A 5-HT$_{2A}$ partial agonist with additional 5-HT$_{1A}$ agonism and dopaminergic effects, a duration of action of 8–20 h may limit potential clinical applications • Studies suggested benefit for pain, existential distress, anxiety, and depressive symptoms among patients with life-threatening illness
DPT[45,46]	• Unscheduled manufactured tryptamine that entered the public eye in the 1960s, subsequently used in a research context by investigators at the Spring Grove State Hospital • Selective 5-HT$_{2A}$ agonist with possible partial agonist activity at the 5-HT$_{1A}$ receptor and monoamine reuptake inhibition properties • Utilized in research in end-of-life distress as well as some studies using PAT to treat patients with alcoholism • Investigated due to its relatively shorter duration of action of 1–2 h making for a more time-effective therapeutic intervention

Nonclassical Psychedelics (not naturally occurring synthetic compounds)

Ketamine	• Schedule 3 dissociative anesthetic with NMDA antagonism and dopaminergic action • May be administered via lozenge, intramuscular injection, intranasally, or by intravenous infusion at regular intervals and subanesthetic doses, with or without concurrent psychotherapy • Racemic esketamine was FDA-approved in 2019 for use in treatment-resistant depression under trade name, Spravato
MDMA	• Schedule 1 substituted amphetamine and empathogen, which stimulates release and reduces reuptake of the monamines serotonin, dopamine, and norepinephrine while also increasing oxytocin levels • Under investigation in Phase 3 clinical trials as adjunct to psychotherapy for the treatment of various anxiety-related conditions, most notably posttraumatic stress disorder receiving with FDA Breakthrough Therapy designation in 2017 • Phase 2 clinical trials suggest benefit in terms of anxiety reduction among patients with life-threatening illness

[a] NB, Schedule I substances are illegal outside the research context in the USA
Adapted from Rosa et al. 2022; with permission[47]

that an "increased acceptance of death usually followed sessions in which the patients' reported deep religious and mystical experiences." Researchers at Spring Grove later sought to find an alternative to LSD that could confer the same effects but minimize the length of sessions. They settled on a compound known as DPT, a shorter-acting serotonergic-based psychedelic. Treating a total of 92 patients utilizing the same protocol, the group found similar significant reductions in measurements of anxiety and depression in patients with terminal cancer.[14]

Following the work at Spring Grove, the scheduling of LSD and other psychedelics as Schedule 1 substances put a halt on clinical research in the United States. Some other European countries continued to use LSD in the psychotherapeutic setting between 1970 and 2010; however, it was not until 2014 that the next clinical trial was published. Led by Peter Gasser at the University of Bern in Switzerland, the group sought to reexamine the safety and efficacy of LSD (200 µg) in 12 patients with life-threatening illness using a double-blind, randomized, placebo-controlled trial design. They found significant reductions in state anxiety that persisted up to 12 months following dosing and a positive trend toward reduction in trait anxiety, with no adverse events reported.[15] In 2022, Holze and colleagues conducted a follow-up phase II, double-blind, randomized controlled trial looking at LSD for anxiety in patients with and without life-threatening illness, finding significant reductions in anxiety and depression that were correlated with the degree of the mystical experience. A single, time-limited, serious adverse event occurred, described as acute but severe anxiety with delusional content.[16]

Psilocybin

In the past decade, the majority of research into PAT has used psilocybin, a natural compound with "classical" psychedelic properties found within the *Psilocybe* genus of mushrooms. Research using psilocybin-assisted therapy has shown significant results for the treatment of treatment-resistant depression, with the FDA (Food and Drug Administration) designating psilocybin as a Breakthrough Therapy and fast-tracking the development and review of its use. To date, there have been 3 randomized, double-blind, placebo-controlled clinical trials that have investigated the use of psilocybin to treat psychological distress in the setting of cancer, and an additional single-arm, open-label study investigating demoralization in patients diagnosed with HIV before the availability of protease inhibitors.

The first study was done by Grob and colleagues in 2011 on 12 patients with anxiety in the setting of advanced-stage cancer. Results from this pilot study showed no adverse events from the administration of moderate-dose psilocybin (0.2 mg/kg) to this patient population, establishing the feasibility and preliminary efficacy of moderate-dose psilocybin in patients with advanced-stage cancer. In addition, analysis of secondary outcomes of anxiety and depression showed significant changes in anxiety at all time points 1 month after dosing and in depression at the 6-month follow-up time point. Based on these results, 2 larger studies were conducted in 2016 by Griffiths and colleagues (51 patients, 0.3–0.45 mg/kg) and Ross and colleagues (29 patients, 0.3 mg/kg). Both studies found significant and sustained improvements in anxiety and depressive symptoms, with the latter showing sustained improvements up to 4.5 years after administration. Associated significant improvements were also seen in measurements of hopelessness, demoralization, quality of life, spiritual well-being, death acceptance, life meaning, and optimism. Furthermore, statistical mediation analysis of treatment outcomes in both studies showed that a mystical-type experience was a mediator in positive therapeutic response, a finding that has been replicated in other studies looking at psychedelics for various psychiatric disorders.[17]

In 2020, Anderson and colleagues completed a single-arm, open-label study investigating the use of a group-based model of psilocybin-assisted therapy in long-term acquired immunodeficiency syndrome survivors experiencing demoralization, defined as "a form of existential suffering characterized by poor coping and a sense of helplessness, hopelessness, and a loss of meaning and purpose in life." Building on the conventional model of PAT, patients attended 8 to 10 group psychotherapy sessions spread throughout the preparation and integration phases in addition to individual preparation and integration. They treated a total of 18 patients with 0.3 to 0.36 mg/kg of psilocybin, with the primary clinical outcome being demoralization as measured by the Demoralization Scale-II. They found clinically meaningful reductions in levels of demoralization at their primary endpoint (3 weeks after dosing), noting an effect size of 0.47 (90% Confidence Interval: 0.21–0.60) with effects sustained for up to 3 months following psilocybin administration. Additionally, no serious adverse events were reported as a result of psilocybin administration.[18]

3,4-methylenedioxymethamphetamine

Most of the clinical research using MDMA-assisted psychotherapy has focused on the treatment of posttraumatic stress disorder, with promising results that led to MDMA being granted a Breakthrough Therapy designation by the FDA. Rather than acting directly at the receptor, MDMA stimulates the release of endogenous monoamines (serotonin, dopamine, norepinephrine) in a mechanism involving the reverse transport of neurotransmitters from inside the cell to the outside. These neurotransmitters are released in elevated quantities relative to baseline, and it is this relative increase, in addition to increasing release of oxytocin, that is thought to mediate its empathogenic effect.[19]

To date, there has been only one study investigating the utility of MDMA in end-of-life anxiety.[20] In a double-blind, placebo-controlled, crossover trial of 18 participants diagnosed with a life-threatening illness, participants were randomized to receive either MDMA or placebo in accordance with the conventional PAT model: three preparation sessions, one dosing session, and three integration sessions. The primary endpoint was changes in STAI-Trait anxiety scores at 1 month, with other secondary endpoints measured at 6 months and 12 months. Results indicated a trend towards a significant reduction in trait anxiety at 1 month, with a P-value of .056; however, the authors note that with the removal of a potential placebo outlier, the results reached significance with a P-value of .0066. Regarding secondary outcomes at 1 month, significant changes were seen on the Post-Traumatic Growth Inventory and Five Factor Mindfulness Questionnaire. Additionally, similar trends toward significance were seen in levels of STAI-State anxiety, depression, sleep, and global functioning. At both the 6-month and 12-month follow-up time points, the changes observed at 1 month were sustained. Regarding specific changes in measures related to LTI-anxiety, subjects showed improvement in fear of death, neutral acceptance, and approach acceptance as measured by the Death Attitudes Profile. The results from this study warrant more rigorous and high-powered studies investigating MDMA in psychiatric symptoms associated with life-threatening illness.

Ketamine

Ketamine has become the first medication with psychedelic properties to become FDA-approved for psychiatric treatment. Ketamine acts as an N-methyl-D-aspartate (NMDA) receptor antagonist, which functions to transiently increase glutamate release throughout the brain. Current research has focused on ketamine's utility in mood disorders, trauma, and addiction. However, there is conflicting evidence as to whether its psychoactive effects mediate its therapeutic benefit.[21] It is important to note that a majority of the ketamine research used the pharmacologic intervention alone without a psychotherapeutic component, a practice that separates the current use of ketamine from the use of other psychedelics described above. Nonetheless, evidence suggests a possible utility for ketamine in quickly treating symptoms of depression and anxiety at the end of life.[22]

All current studies investigating ketamine's use in palliative care looked at the effectiveness of ketamine alone without psychotherapeutic interventions. In one of the first studies, patients in hospice care were given 0.5 mg/kg of oral ketamine daily for 28 days. They found significant and rapid reductions in levels of depression and anxiety among patients.[23] Two retrospective analyses looking at psychological changes in hospitalized palliative patients who received various dosing regimens of ketamine found significant improvements in anxiety and well-being.[24,25] There have been 4 randomized clinical trials looking at a single dose of IV ketamine (0.25–0.5 mg/kg) in patients with serious illness, 3 of which occurred intraoperatively during cancer-related procedures. All showed significant improvements in depression and suicidality lasting up to 3 days, with one showing significant improvements up to 1 month after dosing.[26] Future studies will hopefully look at utilizing ketamine-assisted psychotherapy in a similar way to PAT, utilizing the acute change in consciousness to create insight, understanding, and meaning during the end of life. Currently, there is one registered clinical trial that is planning to investigate this in patients with serious illness, adopting the conventional PAT model of preparation, dosing, and integration (NCT05214417).

Cannabis

The acceptance of medical cannabis among patients with serious illnesses is increasing among the public and healthcare providers alike. An increasing number of states have created laws allowing either medical or both medical and recreational use, despite it still being federally illegal. In 2020, a study noted a 75% increase in cannabis use among people aged 65 years and older from 2015 to 2018. This increase in usage was mainly driven by seniors with comorbid conditions.

Marijuana (*Cannabis sativa*) and hemp (*C sativa* cultivars) both contain the cannabinoids delta-9-tetrahydrocannabinol (THC) and cannabidiol (CBD). THC is the compound associated with psychoactive effects; hemp contains 0.3% compared with the average 15% or greater found in marijuana plants in the United States.[27] Activation of THC on the CB1 and CB2 receptors of the endocannabinoid system has pain-modulatory and psychoactive effects, with CB1 mainly in the central nervous system and CB2 mainly in the peripheral nervous system and immune tissues. CBD is capable of inhibiting the binding of THC to CB1 receptors and has gained popularity due to its non-psychoactive properties, as well as its potential to alleviate symptoms of insomnia, anxiety, pain, social anxiety disorder, and schizophrenia.[28–30] There is also growing evidence for medical cannabis in the treatment of posttraumatic stress disorder.[31]

Although its clinical use is increasing, the medical evidence surrounding the use of cannabis for symptom management remains mixed. Providers caring for older adults with serious illnesses should therefore be familiar with the current evidence regarding its use and potential side effects.[32] Some literature supports the use of cannabis for neuropsychiatric symptoms such as agitation and aggression, which can be seen in patients with dementia, as well as for pain.[33] This could potentially make cannabis an attractive alternative to antipsychotics and opioids, which have unfavorable side effects for older adults. One study using dronabinol (an oral synthetic THC) showed improvement in neuropsychiatric symptoms and appetite in patients with dementia, with low adverse side effects.[34] However, another study that used Namisol (made from plant-based THC) did not show improvement in quality of life or symptoms.[33] A recent review of studies looking at mental health comorbidities reported by older cannabis users (both medical and recreational) found that short-term, low-dose THC medical cannabis use does not seem to carry significant risk of serious cognitive side effects. However, it is suggested that prolonged use may be detrimental to mental health and cognition.[30] However, lack of evidence for dosing of plant-based cannabis complicates recommendations for medical use. Overall, the benefit of treating dementia symptoms with cannabinoids requires further study.

Two small RCTs failed to demonstrate any efficacy of cannabis in treating motor symptoms in patients with Parkinson's disease; however, with suggested improvements in their quality-of-life perception of nonmotor symptoms. A study conducted in 1982 comparing the efficacy of THC to prochlorperazine for treatment of nausea and vomiting in patients with cancer found no difference in the reduction of nausea and vomiting in older adults.[35] Moreover, cannabinoids that are metabolized through the CP450 (CYP3A4, CYP2C9) system can result in drug interactions, which are commonly used in the elderly population, and hence may require an adjustment of medications when used concomitantly.[27,33,36] Older adults are at risk for more adverse outcomes secondary to age-related changes in drug metabolism, organ function, and polypharmacy (**Table 2**).

Especially for THC in high concentrations, cannabis can increase the risk of falls in the elderly owing to its adverse effects on coordination and cognition. Adverse outcomes can include psychosis, delusions, impaired memory, dizziness, muscle relaxation, apathy, sedation, slowed digestion, and hyperemesis in high-potency THC preparations. Products such as full extract cannabis oil (50%–75% THC) and Rick Simpson Oil (60%–90% THC) that contain high-THC concentrations are often promoted to patients and families as a treatment of cancer and other illnesses, yet there is insufficient reliable evidence to support such claims. It is also important to screen elderly regular cannabis users for alcohol use due to a positive correlation between alcohol consumption and cannabis use in people aged older than 50 years.[37]

SUMMARY

Although the current model of palliative care has significantly improved the quality of life in patients with serious illness, pharmacologic interventions for psychological distress at the end of life remain limited despite it being among the most debilitating symptoms in palliative patients. This is largely due to the multidimensional nature of psychological distress in this population, encompassing both physical symptom burden and existential distress. Data surrounding the approved pharmacotherapies used to treat end-of-life distress has shown mixed efficacy.[8,9] Therapeutic interventions such as meaning-centered psychotherapy and dignity therapy have been found to be effective in addressing psychological distress at the end of life, centered around evidence supporting the notion that existential distress is grounded in loss of meaning in one's life; however, manualized therapies often take time, and there remains a need for quick and effective pharmacologic interventions.[12,38]

PAT offers a novel tool to accentuate the therapeutic process of creating meaning amid the loss of self (functionality, relationships, identity, and so forth) that inevitably occurs at the end of life.[11] Research indicates that existential distress is rooted in issues with meaning, purpose, and connection that "lie at the very center of the existential crisis that is terminal illness."[6] Current models of palliative care address these needs through a generalist/specialist model that ideally integrates mental health and

Table 2
Drug–drug interactions with cannabis[48,49,50]

Medication	Interaction	Notes
Warfarin	THC and CBD increase warfarin levels	Increased INR
Theophylline	Inhaled cannabis can decrease drug levels	
Clobazam	CBD increase clobazam levels[51]	
CNS depressant	Cannabis has additive CNS depressant effect	Alcohol increases THC; CBD can alter metabolism of benzodiazepines
Ca channel blocker	Cannabis can increase serum concentrations	THC can induce a cardiovascular stress response that can elevate cardiac oxygen consumption while reducing blood flow in coronary arteries; potentiating hypotension
Amiodarone	Increase THC levels	
Antidepressants	Cannabis can increase serum concentrations of SSRI, SNRI, TCA	
Statins	CBD inhibits several of the liver enzymes which are necessary for breaking down statins	
Rifampin	Decreases effect of CBD	
Antibiotics	Risk of altering metabolization of antibiotics	Clarithromycin and erythromycin can block the liver enzymes that process CBD
Antifungals	Risk of altering metabolization of antifungal	Ketoconazole and itraconazole can block the liver enzymes that process CBD
Morphine	CBD can decrease metabolism of morphine	
Antiretroviral	Cannabis can inhibit the activity of enzymes that metabolize and eliminate antiretroviral therapies from the body[52]	Can result in higher concentrations of ART drugs in the body
Immunosuppressant	CBD can increase the blood levels of immunosuppressants such as tacrolimus and cyclosporine	
Oral hypoglycemic	May have an additive blood glucose lowering effect with hypoglycemic medications	

spiritual care professionals. Yet, in many patients, psychosocial and/or spiritual needs remain under-addressed, and novel therapeutic tools are needed.[39] Although the mechanism of action of PAT has yet to be clearly elucidated, data suggests their efficacy to be rooted in the cultivation of an altered state of consciousness that may help facilitate the therapeutic process of meaning-making through situational acceptance, reprioritization of values, and recontextualization of the self in light of functional losses.[11]

As opposed to PAT, the use of ketamine in palliative care has focused on the medication itself, without paired psychotherapeutic processes. The available data supports ketamine as an intervention for quick and effective psychiatric symptom management in a frequently treatment-resistant population, arguably providing the fastest psychological symptom relief as compared with all current interventions. However, the sustainability of its effect remains in question. It also remains unclear if and how ketamine's psychoactive properties relate to its therapeutic efficacy and how its pain management abilities play a role in alleviating psychological distress in patients with a high symptom burden. Similarly, some evidence supports a possible role for cannabis as an intervention for quick and effective symptom relief with a favorable side effect profile as compared with the current standard of treatment. However, the current cannabis studies are inconsistent, suggesting mixed efficacy. As such, more rigorous evidence is needed on both ketamine and cannabis in elderly patients in palliative care before supporting adoption into clinical practice. Of note, similar to ketamine, there is emerging discussion of cannabis-assisted psychotherapy within community treatment practices, suggesting a possible role for cannabis augmenting therapy in a manner like PAT. However, there is currently no scientific evidence investigating this model of therapeutic cannabis use as an intervention for psychological distress at the end of life.

It is important to note the current contraindications to these therapies despite their promise. All interventions that produce an acute change in consciousness carry a risk of psychosis, and as such, having a personal or family history of schizophrenia-spectrum disorders is a contraindication to use. For PAT and ketamine, a majority of research studies include bipolar in the list of contraindicated diagnoses; however, data is emerging that shows the risk of PAT exacerbating psychosis in patients with a personal or family history of bipolar disorder may be lower than expected.[40] Similarly, data is also emerging supporting the safety and efficacy of ketamine in treating bipolar depression.[41] Conversely, data shows that the use of cannabis with high-THC content may exacerbate the risk of psychosis in predisposed individuals and thus should be avoided in all patients with a personal or family history of psychosis.[42] From a medical standpoint, all of the aforementioned pharmacotherapies cause acute increases in blood pressure and heart rate, and as such, careful cardiovascular screening (history, electrocardiogram, stress test) is necessary for individuals with cardiovascular disease.[43]

Although data surrounding the safety and tolerability of cannabis in the elderly is growing with legalization, there remains a scarcity of data on the safety, acceptability, and tolerability of psychedelics in patients aged older than 65 years, with only a small minority of participants in psychedelic research trials within this age range.[44] Given that a majority of serious illness patients fall within this age range, more research is needed before psychedelic-based therapies can be implemented in palliative care. As data continues to emerge, the utility of these novel psychoactive treatment modalities for older adults in palliative care will continue to be evaluated; however, the current data support the potential use of PAT and ketamine as safe and effective interventions in addressing the multidimensional nature of end-of-life distress in elderly patients in palliative care. Although some data supports the potential use of cannabis for symptom relief, the data is mixed, and as such, further research is needed before conclusions can be drawn on its utility in this population.

CLINICS CARE POINTS

- Psychological distress is a multidimensional phenomenon in elderly patients in palliative care for which available interventions are limited.
- PAT may help treat existential distress by facilitating the process of meaning-making.
- Ketamine may provide quick and effective relief from depression and anxiety in a population where time is limited.
- Some evidence suggests that cannabis may provide quick and effective relief from physical symptom burden as well as depression and anxiety; however, the data is inconclusive.

DISCLOSURE

Y. Beaussant's research focuses on developing and assessing psychedelic-assisted therapies in patients with serious illness. He received philanthropic research funding from the Oppenheimer Family Psychosocial Oncology and Palliative Care Research Grants, Carey and Claudia Turnbull Family Foundation, Heffter Research Institute, United States, George Sarlo Foundation, United States, RiverStyx Foundation, Council on Spiritual Practices Fund at the San Francisco Foundation, Nikean Foundation, and Jack Smith, as well research grants from Sunstone Therapies. K. Nigam is an independent contractor for Acuta Capital Partners, a healthcare financial investment group, and provides independent, psychopharmacology-related consulting services. K. Nigam only receives compensation for professional consultations and has no stake in the company or its investments.

REFERENCES

1. Issues C on ADAKE of L, Medicine I of. Epidemiology of Serious Illness and High Utilization of Health Care. National Academies Press (US); 2015. Available at: https://www.ncbi.nlm.nih.gov/books/NBK285684/. Accessed January 12, 2023.
2. Temel JS, Greer JA, Muzikansky A, et al. Early palliative care for patients with metastatic non–small-cell lung cancer. N Engl J Med 2010;363(8):733–42.
3. Kozlov E, Cai A, Sirey JA, et al. Identifying palliative care needs among older adults in nonclinical settings. Am J Hosp Palliat Care 2018;35(12):1477–82.
4. Rostoft S, Thomas MJ, Slaaen M, et al. The effect of age on specialized palliative care use in the last year of life for patients who die of cancer: a nationwide study from Norway. J Geriatr Oncol 2022;13(8):1103–10.
5. Ljuslin M, Nigam K, Sholevar R, et al. Psychedelic-assisted therapies in patients with serious illness: opportunities and challenges. Psychiatr Ann 2022;52(9):359–64.
6. McClain CS, Rosenfeld B, Breitbart W. Effect of spiritual well-being on end-of-life despair in terminally-ill cancer patients. Lancet 2003;361(9369):1603–7.
7. Stroebe MS, Stroebe W. The mortality of bereavement: a review. In: Stroebe MS, Stroebe W, Hansson RO, editors. Handbook of bereavement: theory, research, and intervention. Cambridge, UK: Cambridge University Press; 1993. p. 175–95. https://doi.org/10.1017/CBO9780511664076.013.

8. Cheer SM, Goa KL. Fluoxetine: a review of its therapeutic potential in the treatment of depression associated with physical illness. Drugs 2001;61(1):81–110.

9. Riblet N, Larson R, Watts BV, et al. Reevaluating the role of antidepressants in cancer-related depression: a systematic review and meta-analysis. Gen Hosp Psychiatr 2014;36(5):466–73.

10. Mystakidou K, Tsilika E, Parpa E, et al. Psychological distress of patients with advanced cancer: influence and contribution of pain severity and pain interference. Cancer Nurs 2006;29(5):400.

11. Beaussant Y, Nigam K. Expending perspectives on the potential for psychedelic-assisted therapies to improve the experience of aging. Am J Geriatr Psychiatry 2023;31(1):54–7.

12. Boston P, Bruce A, Schreiber R. Existential suffering in the palliative care setting: an integrated literature review. J Pain Symptom Manage 2011;41(3):604–18.

13. Knudsen GM. Sustained effects of single doses of classical psychedelics in humans. Neuropsychopharmacology 2023;48(1):145–50.

14. Bossis A, Grob CS, Grigsby J. Utility of psychedelics in the treatment of psycho-spiritual and existential distress in palliative care. NY, USA: Guilford Publications; 2021.

15. Gasser P, Holstein D, Michel Y, et al. Safety and efficacy of lysergic acid diethylamide-assisted psychotherapy for anxiety associated with life-threatening diseases. J Nerv Ment Dis 2014;202(7):513–20.

16. Holze F, Gasser P, Müller F, et al. Lysergic acid diethylamide–assisted therapy in patients with anxiety with and without a life-threatening illness: a randomized, double-blind, placebo-controlled phase II study. Biol Psychiatry 2022;0(0). https://doi.org/10.1016/j.biopsych.2022.08.025.

17. Yaden DB, Griffiths RR. The subjective effects of psychedelics are necessary for their enduring therapeutic effects. ACS Pharmacol Transl Sci 2021;4(2):568–72.

18. Anderson BT, Danforth A, Daroff PR, et al. Psilocybin-assisted group therapy for demoralized older long-term AIDS survivor men: an open-label safety and feasibility pilot study. EClinicalMedicine 2020;27:100538.

19. Rudnick G, Wall SC. The molecular mechanism of "ecstasy" [3,4-methylenedioxy-methamphetamine (MDMA)]: serotonin transporters are targets for MDMA-induced serotonin release. Proc Natl Acad Sci 1992;89(5):1817–21.

20. Wolfson PE, Andries J, Feduccia AA, et al. MDMA-assisted psychotherapy for treatment of anxiety and other psychological distress related to life-threatening illnesses: a randomized pilot study. Sci Rep 2020;10(1):20442.

21. Ballard ED, Zarate CA. The role of dissociation in ketamine's antidepressant effects. Nat Commun 2020;11(1):6431.

22. Rothberg RL, Azhari N, Haug NA, et al. Mystical-type experiences occasioned by ketamine mediate its impact on at-risk drinking: results from a randomized, controlled trial. J Psychopharmacol 2021;35(2):150–8.

23. Irwin SA, Iglewicz A, Nelesen RA, et al. Daily oral ketamine for the treatment of depression and anxiety in patients receiving hospice care: a 28-day open-label proof-of-concept trial. J Palliat Med 2013;16(8):958–65.

24. Falk E, Schlieper D, van Caster P, et al. A rapid positive influence of S-ketamine on the anxiety of patients in palliative care: a retrospective pilot study. BMC Palliat Care 2020;19(1):1.

25. Iglewicz A, Morrison K, Nelesen RA, et al. Ketamine for the treatment of depression in patients receiving hospice care: a retrospective medical record review of thirty-one cases. Psychosomatics 2015;56(4):329–37.

26. Schimmel N, Breeksema JJ, Smith-Apeldoorn SY, et al. Psychedelics for the treatment of depression, anxiety, and existential distress in patients with a terminal illness: a systematic review. Psychopharmacology (Berl) 2022;239(1):15–33.

27. Cash MC, Cunnane K, Fan C, et al. Mapping cannabis potency in medical and recreational programs in the United States. PLoS One 2020;15(3):e0230167.

28. Noel C. Evidence for the use of "medical marijuana" in psychiatric and neurologic disorders. Ment Health Clin 2017;7(1):29–38.

29. Lucas CJ, Galettis P, Schneider J. The pharmacokinetics and the pharmacodynamics of cannabinoids. Br J Clin Pharmacol 2018;84(11):2477–82.

30. Vacaflor BE, Beauchet O, Jarvis GE, et al. Mental health and cognition in older cannabis users: a review. Can Geriatr J 2020;23(3):242–9.

31. Walsh Z, Gonzalez R, Crosby K, et al. Medical cannabis and mental health: a guided systematic review. Clin Psychol Rev 2017;51:15–29.

32. Winston H. Cannabis in the geriatric population. In: Riggs P, Thant T, editors. Cannabis in psychiatric practice: a practical guide. Psychiatry update. NY, USA: Springer International Publishing; 2022. p. 179–89. https://doi.org/10.1007/978-3-031-04874-6_16.

33. Ahmed AIA, van den Elsen GAH, Colbers A, et al. Safety, pharmacodynamics, and pharmacokinetics of multiple oral doses of delta-9-tetrahydrocannabinol in older persons with dementia. Psychopharmacology (Berl) 2015;232(14):2587–95.

34. Kuharic DB, Markovic D, Brkovic T, et al. Cannabinoids for the treatment of dementia. Cochrane Database Syst Rev 2021;(9). https://doi.org/10.1002/14651858.CD012820.pub2.

35. Ungerleider JT, Andrysiak T, Fairbanks L, et al. Cannabis and cancer chemotherapy: a comparison of oral delta-9-THC and prochlorperazine. Cancer 1982;50(4):636–45.

36. Worster B, Hajjar ER, Handley N. Cannabis use in patients with cancer: a clinical review. JCO Oncol Pract 2022;18(11):743–9.

37. Han BH, Palamar JJ. Trends in cannabis use among older adults in the United States, 2015-2018. JAMA Intern Med 2020;180(4):609–11.

38. Breitbart W, Pessin H, Rosenfeld B, et al. Individual meaning-centered psychotherapy for the treatment of psychological and existential distress: a randomized controlled trial in patients with advanced cancer. Cancer 2018;124(15):3231–9.

39. Periyakoil VS, Gunten CF von, Fischer S, et al. Generalist versus specialist palliative medicine. J Palliat Med 2022;25(2):193–9.

40. Gard DE, Pleet MM, Bradley ER, et al. Evaluating the risk of psilocybin for the treatment of bipolar depression: a review of the research literature and published case studies. J Affect Disord Rep 2021;6:100240.

41. Wilkowska A, Szałach Ł, Cubała WJ. Ketamine in bipolar disorder: a review. Neuropsychiatr Dis Treat 2020;16:2707–17.

42. Sideli L, Quigley H, La Cascia C, et al. Cannabis use and the risk for psychosis and affective disorders. J Dual Diagn 2020;16(1):22–42.

43. Frecska E. Therapeutic guidelines: dangers and contra-indications in therapeutic applications of hallucinogens. In: Roberts T, Winkelman M, editors. Psychedelic Medicine. CT, USA: Praeger; 2007. p. 69–95.

44. Johnston CB, Mangini M, Grob C, et al. The safety and efficacy of psychedelic-assisted therapies for older adults: knowns and unknowns. Am J Geriatr Psychiatry 2022. https://doi.org/10.1016/j.jagp.2022.08.007.

45. Fantegrossi WE, Reissig CJ, Katz EB, et al. Hallucinogen-like effects of N,N-dipropyltryptamine (DPT): possible mediation by serotonin 5-HT1A and 5-HT2A receptors in rodents. Pharmacol Biochem Behav 2008;88(3):358–65.

46. Rhead JC, Soskin RA, Turek I, et al. Psychedelic drug (DPT)-assisted psychotherapy with alcoholics: a controlled study. J Psychedelic Drugs 1977;9:287–300.

47. Rosa WE, Sager Z, Miller M, et al. Top ten tips palliative care clinicians should know about psychedelic-assisted therapy in the context of serious illness. J Palliat Med 2022;25(8):1273–81.

48. Antoniou T, Bodkin J, Ho JM-W, et al. Drug interactions with cannabinoids. CMJA 2020;192(9):E206.

49. Lopera VR, Rodríguez A, Amariles P. Clinical relevance of drug interactions with cannabis: A systematic review. J Clin Med 2022;11(5):1154.

50. Davis M. Cannabinoid-Based Medicine: Pharmacology and Drug Interactions. In: Cannabis and Cannabinoid-Based Medicines in Cancer Care. Cham: Springer; 2022. p. 41–89.

51. Geffrey AL, Pollack SF, Bruno PL, Thiele EA. Drug–drug interaction between clobazam and cannabidiol in children with refractory epilepsy. Epilepsia 2015;56(8):1246–51.

52. Mills AN, Nichols MA, Davenport E. Chronic pain and medical cannabis: Narrative review and practice considerations in persons living with HIV. J Am Coll Clin Pharm 2022;5(3):342–53.

Early Palliative Care for the Geriatric Patient with Cancer

Colleen Carroll, APRN-CNP[a],
Lori Ruder, DNP, APRN-CNP, AGACNP-BC, ACHPN[a],
Christine Miklosovic, RN-BSN, CHPCA[a], Rev. Matthew Bauhof, MDiv[a],
Lauren Chiec, MD[b], Cynthia Owusu, MD, MS[b],
Kimberly A. Curseen, MD, FAAHPM[c], Mona Gupta, MD, AGSF, FAAHPM[d],*

KEYWORDS

- Early palliative care • Geriatric cancer • Symptom management

KEY POINTS

- Older adults with cancer often have a multitude of physical and psychosocial needs that may benefit from early implementation of palliative care.
- Older adults with cancer have unique metabolic and pharmacologic considerations that may impact care.
- A thorough assessment of both palliative and geriatric domains may help to identify problems unique to the older adult with cancer and help to address these needs in a timely manner.
- Multidisciplinary involvement is the key to achieving adequate palliative care management for many older adults in the oncology space.

[a] Division of Solid Tumor Oncology, Supportive and Palliative Oncology, University Hospitals Seidman Cancer Center, 11100 Euclid Avenue, Lakeside Suite 1200, Mailstop LKS 5079, Cleveland, OH 44106, USA; [b] Division of Solid Tumor Oncology, Case Western Reserve University School of Medicine, University Hospitals Seidman Cancer Center, 11100 Euclid Avenue, Lakeside Suite 1200, Mailstop LKS 5079, Cleveland, OH 44106, USA; [c] Division of Palliative Care, Department of Family Preventative Medicine, Emory School of Medicine, 1365 Clifton NE, Atlanta, GA 30322, USA; [d] Division of Solid Tumor Oncology, Supportive and Palliative Oncology, Case Western Reserve University School of Medicine, University Hospitals Seidman Cancer Center, 11100 Euclid Avenue, Lakeside Suite 1200, Mailstop LKS 5079, Cleveland, OH 44106, USA
* Corresponding author. University Hospitals Seidman Cancer Center, 11100 Euclid Avenue, Lakeside Suite 1200, Mailstop LKS 5079, Cleveland, OH 44106.
E-mail address: Mona.Gupta@UHHospitals.org

Clin Geriatr Med 39 (2023) 437–448
https://doi.org/10.1016/j.cger.2023.04.005
0749-0690/23/© 2023 Elsevier Inc. All rights reserved.
geriatric.theclinics.com

BACKGROUND

Cancer is known to be a disease that disproportionally affects older adults with numerous disease burdens and treatment side effects that can influence a patient's quality of life, ranging from physical discomfort to complex psychosocial symptoms.[1] When combined with aging, which has an independent list of considerations, addressing the quality of life of older adults living with cancer is a growing interest in the medical field.[2] Research indicates that palliative care for patients living with cancer can help to achieve adequate symptom management, allow patients and families to feel supported, and in some instances, correlates with prolonged survival.[3] The timely implementation of palliative care can also allow for adequate comfort measures and support at the end of life.[4] In a study done by Hannon, older adults often verbalized wishing they were referred to palliative care sooner.[4] This article explores the importance of early integration of palliative care for older adults with cancer.

CARE DELIVERY CONSIDERATIONS

It is important to note that palliative care may be delivered to patients in a multitude of ways and settings. Although variable and dependent on the institution, palliative care is often delivered by a multidisciplinary team approach. Larger hospital systems may have both inpatient and outpatient palliative care teams consisting of physicians, advanced practice providers, nurses, social workers, counselors, and supportive therapies (such as music, art, and spiritual care). There are also community-based programs that deliver care in the home and in facilities. Based on the patient's needs, a palliative care team can follow the patient throughout their cancer journey. Having the palliative care team involved affords oncology and geriatric providers the opportunity to defer the primary symptom management responsibility to trained palliative care teams, leaving room for collaboration and the development of the best plan of care for the patient. This is especially important given the elderly are often more prone to swift, symptom-related decline.[5] There is still considerable confusion concerning the understanding of the scope of palliative care, among many patients, families, and referring providers. They may be unaware of palliative care's role in symptom management outside of end-of-life care and there can be confusion with hospice care, which is comfort-based care that is exclusively provided to the terminally ill in the final stages of life. Continued widespread education regarding palliative care and its benefit will allow more individuals to gain access to this type of care.

Primary palliative care is symptom-based, quality-of-life focused care delivered by oncologists and geriatricians. Specialty palliative care is directly provided by the palliative care team. It is recognized that many aspects of palliative care delivery may occur through primary care providers, reserving specialty-level referrals for more complex assessments and management. When referral to a palliative care specialist is not possible, the responsibility of symptom management lies with the oncology and geriatric medicine teams caring for the respective patient. This highlights the importance of oncologists having training in both primary palliative care and geriatric principles so that the unique needs of these patients can be met. This also highlights the need for improved strategies to identify which patients may benefit most from early specialty level referrals. Continuing research on this is needed to identify gaps of care for geriatric patients with cancer. For the purpose of this article, delivery of palliative care or "referral" to palliative care can refer to care from a primary palliative care provider as well as from a palliative care specialist.

COMBINED ASSESSMENT APPROACH

A key argument for early referral of palliative care for this population is to allow for timely geriatric *and* palliative care assessments, with intentional overlap, to best serve the patient. A purposeful component of a thorough, combined assessment is evaluating the patient's current symptoms and multidimensional geriatric assessment that includes functional status evaluation. The importance of integrating palliative care with geriatric assessment is that it will help to detect problems not routinely identified that would otherwise adversely impact both oncology care and palliative care. Of particular relevance for evaluation is the patient's present level of and risk for worsening frailty. Frailty can be defined as declining physical reserve that predisposes one to adverse health events.[6] Although frailty can be both physical (fatigue, low activity, weakness, weight loss, slow gait) and a result of deficit accumulation (impacted by cumulative medical comorbidities), it is linked to overall decline and increasing vulnerability to poor cancer-related outcomes.[2] It is important to consider frailty as a spectrum. Patients at risk for frailty, or "pre-frailty," may be identified through a variety of assessment domains.[6] Discussing these findings can allow for appropriate care planning and education of the patient, as acute illness and cancer-related complications may cause worsening medical vulnerability for these older adults, known as secondary frailty (**Fig. 1**).[6]

Frailty is an important consideration in the setting of a new or recurrent malignancy. With that in mind, a growing body of research indicates that patients who score poorly on the comprehensive geriatric assessment (CGA), or on pre-geriatric assessment screening tools such as the G8 assessment tool, which identifies elderly patients

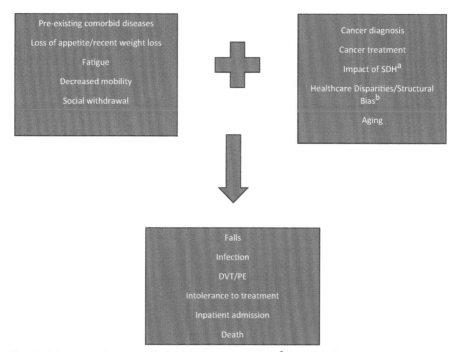

Fig. 1. Adverse pathway of frail elderly cancer adult.[6] [a] Social determinants of health. [b] Health care disparities/structural bias: effects of environmental inequities, structural and institution racism, clinician bias, poverty, geographic discrimination.

with cancer who could benefit from the CGA, are also at higher risk for cancer treatment-related toxicities and complications.[5] Side effects such as nausea, peripheral neuropathy, and fatigue can be anticipated preemptively and closely managed. Education and decision-making regarding risks, prevention, and treatments for therapy-related complications, such as infection or venous thromboembolism (VTE), can be completed before the onset of any treatment, whether the therapy has curative, disease stabilization, or palliative intent.

By identifying and pairing commonalities in geriatric and palliative care assessments, risks can be assessed and interventions can be implemented to address all components. Using the National Consensus Project for Quality Palliative Care recommended palliative care domains and interventions, the International Society of Geriatric Oncology recommended geriatric assessment domains, information obtained from the Geriatric Assessment-Driven Intervention and Chemotherapy Toxic Effects in Older Adults with Cancer trial, and the multidisciplinary team of authors' professional knowledge and experience, a table was created. The table is designed to identify the commonalities in assessment domains, common challenges for the geriatric oncology patient, and the palliative care team response (**Table 1**).[7–9]

An example using both geriatrics and palliative care assessment domains would be through identifying a patient with a high fall risk. The CGA identifies and quantifies the risk through the functional status domain, whereas the palliative care assessment identifies the symptoms contributing to the high falls risk status. This would be especially important for a patient who may be expected to receive treatment with a high incidence of causing peripheral neuropathy, such as taxanes, platinums, and vinca alkaloids.[10] The numbness, tingling, and burning pain of the extremities associated with peripheral neuropathy are correlated with a higher risk for falls.[11] A patient who, in early assessments, is already exemplifying frailty with ongoing weight loss and taste changes may then be identified as a poor candidate for highly emetogenic treatments, such as the combination of anthracycline and cyclophosphamide, or cisplatin.[12] This information can be presented to the patient and family in a timely manner, which gives the patient the necessary knowledge to make important decisions. If a patient opts to pursue any kind of disease-modifying or stabilizing treatment, the palliative care assessment can be used as a framework to develop a symptom management plan that may prevent or mitigate further decline.

Another example of the presentation of frailty in older adults in the oncology space is cancer cachexia, a syndrome with combined manifestations such as weight loss, muscle wasting, and decline in physical function in the setting of cancer.[1] Older adults are more prone to this syndrome than younger adults in the cancer population with research showing a significant correlation between cancer cachexia with poor outcomes and decreased quality of life.[1] Older adults may benefit from tracking weight and dietary interventions, especially those who suffer from weight loss leading up to their diagnosis, to allow for early management.

These combined assessment factors play a significant role in determining the patient's course of treatment as well as adding the anticipatory guidelines for supportive care. This also allows for an educational opportunity with patients and families regarding the tenuous nature of frailty. Often, older adults may present with good functional status at the onset of the disease but then decline suddenly with treatment. Although research on this is limited, implementation of in-depth geriatric and palliative care assessments on diagnosis may allow for early discussion of these key findings. It also presents an opportunity for early education regarding how to manage symptoms at home. Weight loss and frailty may also prompt serious illness discussion and advance care planning secondary to their adverse effects on prognosis. When

Table 1
Palliative care areas of impact for geriatric cancer patients

Palliative Care Domain	Geriatric Assessment Domain	Common Challenges in Geriatric Oncology	Palliative Care Response
Structure and processes of care	Structure and Processes of care	• Transfers to and from home and inpatient care centers • Transportation difficulties • Complex and frequent testing and treatment visits • Pause in cancer treatment	• Patient and family education • Multidisciplinary team support; social work involvement • May allow for improved access to care and communication between care teams
Physical aspects of care	Functional status	• Frailty, low reserve • Functional status impacts ability to receive treatment • Fall risks	• Comprehensive assessment, facilitate complex decision-making discussions, referral to rehabilitation services
	Comorbidities Polypharmacy	• Altered organ function; increased risk of toxicity from common medications • Lengthy medication lists	• Early medication reconciliation, potential simplifying of medication list to minimize risk (targeted de-prescribing in collaboration with patient primary care and specialist)
	Nutrition Clinical symptoms	• Taste and appetite changes • Pain • Nausea • Fatigue • Dyspnea • Constipation/diarrhea • Anxiety, depression • Cognitive decline	• Referral to nutrition services • Complex symptom management

(continued on next page)

Table 1 (continued)			
Palliative Care Domain	Geriatric Assessment Domain	Common Challenges in Geriatric Oncology	Palliative Care Response
Psychologic and psychiatric aspects of care	Psychological/mental health status	• Mood changes, risk of depression and anxiety	• Pharmacologic and non-pharmacologic management of mood changes • Psychological assessment and counseling
	Cognition	• Presence of cognitive impairment • Risk for delirium • Decision-making capacity unclear	• Early advance care planning • Capacity assessment • Social work assessment and resource question
Social aspects of care	Social activity and support	• Limited social support • Caregiver burnout • Social determinants of health; food/housing insecurity	• Multidisciplinary support for patient and family; referral to community resources • Social work referral
Spiritual and religious aspects of care	Spiritual well-being	• Spiritual and existential crises related to aging and diagnosis	• Involvement of chaplain and spiritual support services: spiritual assessment and counseling • Assistance with maintaining connection to spiritual community
Cultural aspects of care	Cultural aspects	• Institutional racism, mistrust • Culture's impact on medical decision-making and communication • Appropriately identifying patient's intersectionality[a]	• Trust building • Identifying and mitigating effects of structural and institutional racism on patient's care through patient advocacy • Developing treatment plans with patients that are sensitive

		to how they experience their intersectionality • Exploration of cultural values and patient's preferences for care and communication • Assist patients to advocate for their goals to their oncology team; facilitating patient wishes based on patient/family value structure
Care of the patient at end of life	• Rapid clinical decline • Limited support to remain safely at home • Symptom management at end of life	• Multidisciplinary care at the end of life, hospice referrals when appropriate • Assessment of caregiver/family stress • Address patient and family resources that could present barriers to patient care at end of life (financial, lack of caregiver, housing insecurity, and so forth)
Caregivers	• Caregiver stress • Lack of access caregiver resources to support patient • Lack of caregiver and or legal surrogate	• Assessment of caregiver stress and multidisciplinary support for caregivers • Assessment of family and caregiver prognostic awareness • Identification of legal surrogates and caregiver • Identification and referral for resources for caregiver support and supplemental patient care
Ethical and legal aspects of care	• Complex family dynamics • Surrogate decision-makers	• Early and ongoing advance care planning and serious illness communication

a Intersectionality: interconnected nature of social categorizations such as race, class, and gender as they apply to a given individual or group, regarded as creating overlapping and interdependent systems of discrimination or disadvantage.

escalation of care is necessary, patients and families may be more prepared to accept this step.[4]

OPPORTUNITY FOR EDUCATION

Early palliative care assessment and implementation also allows an opportunity to educate the patient and family on possible future outcomes. Both cancer and advanced age can be considered life-limiting and are often even more so in combination.[2] It is important to assess the patient and family's comfort level regarding prognosis, goals of care, and possible adverse outcomes. If a patient wishes to be informed and prepared for the future, this allows time for advance care planning discussions. A vital piece of this is giving the patient the option to complete advance directive documents, whereas they are feeling well enough to engage in the discussions needed to complete this paperwork. This, in turn, opens opportunities for the patient to voice priorities so that goals of care can be aligned with their hopes, values, and wishes. The patient may benefit from having these conversations initiated on diagnosis and continued throughout cancer treatment, rather than strictly when the end of life is imminent. Current qualitative research indicates that patients and families appreciate being informed regarding the status of their cancer and possible outcomes, just as they prefer to have ample time to prepare for realistic outcomes.[2]

Interdisciplinary Involvement

Another beneficial factor that stems from timely geriatric and palliative evaluation is the early inclusion of members of the multidisciplinary team. There are complex social and financial issues linked often to aging. Older adults may have limited income. They may be dealing with the stress of identifying housing and care level needs, along with the cost of medical bills, prescriptions, and nutrient-dense foods. This can be overwhelming when factoring in the rising costs of cancer care.[1] In addition, older adults are historically prone to falls and a loss of independence, which can happen more hastily with the symptoms and burdens of cancer treatment. This becomes difficult to monitor as, often, cancer treatment may pause when a patient falls or is admitted to a skilled nursing facility, and ongoing transportation issues arise, as many older adults may not be comfortable with or fit to drive. Given the compound stress of these factors, it is understood that older adults living with cancer are more prone to depression and anxiety, which can be promptly screened for and addressed as via palliative care assessment.[1]

The condition of the older adult may decline due to cancer symptoms or treatment-related side effects, compounded with natural aging. This may warrant the older adult having help at home, should that be a safe possibility. This requires careful assessment and education of the patient and family. Palliative care often works closely with social workers to address these needs early and often to ensure the safest care for the patient and allow for advance care planning documents to be organized, whereas the older adult is well enough to participate. Social workers are also trained to assist in the discussion and process of advance care planning, a critical component to care of the older adult with cancer. They can also provide resources to manage the social determents of health that impact patient ability to maintain function and participate in care.

An imperative aspect of symptom management with the geriatric patient with cancer is nutrition, as nausea and loss of appetite are both frequently associated with cancer treatment. Metabolic and taste changes are common findings among the aging population.[4] Identifying the specific needs of these patients through early palliative care implementation can allow for the early introduction of registered dietician services. Having this qualified member of the interdisciplinary team involved can help to address these concerns, allowing for improved quality of life, and often, tolerance to treatment.[1] In the same respect, physical and occupational therapists are vital members of the supportive care team that can help to build and maintain strength and function. Speech therapists are important for evaluating safe swallowing and digestion through an older adult's cancer journey. This is imperative for older adults dealing with cancers of the gastrointestinal tract, as well as malignancies of the head and neck, as the tumors themselves may impair basic digestive functioning.

An important, often undertreated effect of these social concerns, and patient care is caregiver burn out. This can be addressed by early palliative care implementation. Older adults living with cancer are often dependent on loved ones for housing, transportation, financial assistance, appointment companions, communication of needs, and emotional support through their experience.[13] Family members and friends often have to rework their lives and priorities to provide adequate care to fulfill the needs and wishes of the patient. Research on the topic indicates that caregiver burnout can lead to an increased risk for caregivers to develop a varied list of comorbidities in the Western world, such as depression or diabetes.[13] Connecting the patient's caregivers to the appropriate community resources early is a key component to establishing consistent and thorough care around the patient, allowing all members of the patient's home caregiving team to feel valued, supported, and holistically well. Although the CGA and palliative care assessment are comprehensive, they are lacking in identifying directly the effects of structural and institutional racism and bias that can impact the way in which care is delivered and received for older adults in minoritized communities. Attention should be paid to supplementing the comprehensive review with appropriate questions and interventions to specifically address the intersectionality of older adults from minoritized background, gender minorities, and with lower social economic status. These assessments should be approached with cultural humility to develop collaborative care plans that meet the needs of the patients and families. More research is needed to understand how to do this effectively.[14]

Given the practice of inquiring about the quality of life, values, goals, and concerns, providers administering palliative care are in a unique position to assess the emotional and spiritual needs of older adults living with cancer. Identifying and discussing these important domains of health and well-being early in an older adult's cancer journey allows for a timely opportunity to include art, music, and spiritual care specialists in the patient and family's care. Although each person's spiritual and emotional needs are unique, older adults living with cancer are universally prone to certain factors that influence these needs. The loss of function and independence, dependence on others, and the approaching end of life all place older adults at higher risk for spiritual distress.[13] Incorporating different holistic modalities and interdisciplinary specialists at the onset of a cancer diagnosis can allow geriatric patients to develop healthy coping mechanisms and feel at peace with their diagnosis and choice of clinical options. Implementing spiritual care may even improve patients' adherence to treatment, which can lead to positive outcomes.[13]

PHARMACOLOGIC CONSIDERATIONS

Involving all aspects of a supportive care team can help to de-prescribe unnecessary medication usage for any patient, particularly patients with cancer, in order to reduce polypharmacy and inappropriate prescribing. It is inevitable, though, between treatment and innumerable possible side effects, that a geriatric patient with cancer will be on multiple medications to help manage their cancer, other comorbidities, and cancer-related symptoms. Another limiting factor in this realm is the limited metabolic reserve of many older adults, along with the decline of liver and kidney function often seen with older adults and any-aged patients with cancer. Palliative care providers will perform medication reconciliations early and often, so that cancer care and palliative care treatment plans can be optimized and delivered safely in collaboration with the patient's primary care provider, along with other specialty providers involved in the patient's care. The American Geriatrics Society Beers Criteria for potentially inappropriate medication use in older adults are a targeted set of evidence-based recommendations specifically for older adults (65 years and older) and it is important to recognize that many medications used to manage cancer-related symptoms (opioids, anticholinergics, benzodiazepines, antipsychotics, and so forth) are included in the lists of medications to avoid or use with caution due to increased risk of adverse effects. It is noted, however, the Beers Criteria provide exceptions for the use of medications in the hospice or palliative care setting.[15] Even with these exceptions, medications must be used with expertise and caution to mitigate harm. Palliative care providers are skilled at using these medications that may benefit multiple cancer-related symptoms. They work with a goal to effectively manage side effects and improve quality of life and tolerance to treatment while reducing pill burden and risk for medication interactions.

Early involvement of palliative care in geriatric patients with cancer allows maximum time to abide by the famous geriatric adage "start low and go slow" in regard to medication initiation and dosing. As it is well known that older adults are underrepresented in clinical trials of cancer therapeutics, the impact of treatments, with respect to response and toxicities, is often less well-understood in this population. Palliative care teams are uniquely skilled in facilitating decision-making discussions when outcomes are uncertain, and early involvement allows for the timely management of toxicities or disease-related complications that may arise.[16] Close monitoring and shared decision-making regarding medication choices provide holistic, patient-centered care so that maximal symptom relief with minimal adverse reactions can be achieved safely and effectively.

SUMMARY

A cancer diagnosis and oncology care plan may be difficult to manage as an older adult. Early integration of combined palliative care and geriatric assessment, used through the framework of cultural humility, may help to identify the complex needs of an older adult living with cancer. Implementation of whole-person, symptom-based care early in an older adult's cancer journey may allow for educated decision-making, increased quality of life, adequate clinical and emotional support for patients and caregivers, and efficient integration of the interdisciplinary team members.[1] With older adults in the oncology space, it is important to consider the factor of frailty, along with changes in metabolism and risk for polypharmacy, which may be best addressed at the onset of an older adult's cancer treatment plan.[15] These concerns may be addressed in a high-quality manner via the delivery of palliative care, allowing for safe and efficient management of cancer-related symptoms and treatment-related side effects. This added support and safety net not only can lead to decreased symptom burden, but may mitigate negative outcomes and allow for prolonged quantity and quality of life.[1] When end-of-life is imminent, this holistic support may help to achieve comfort and peace in death.[2] Continued research in this domain may help to further education and palliative care resources for older adults with cancer.

CLINICS CARE POINTS

- Standardized assessments including both geriatric and palliative care domains should be utilized for all older adults with cancer to guide optimal supportive interventions.
- Interdisciplinary team involvement is crucial to providing comprehensive palliative care to older adults with cancer.
- Early involvement of palliative care for older adults with cancer may lead to improved outcomes and allows for ongoing assessments and intervention throughout a patient's disease course

DISCLOSURE

The authors have nothing to disclose.

REFERENCES

1. Nipp R, Subbiah I, Loscalzo M. Convergence of geriatrics and palliative care to deliver personalized supportive care for older adults with cancer. J Clin Oncol 2021;39(19):2185–94.
2. Parajuli J, Tark A, Joa YL, et al. Barries to palliative and hospice care utilization in older adults with cancer: a systematic review. J Geriatr Oncol 2020;11(1):8–20.
3. Temel JS, Greer JA, Muzikansky A, et al. Early palliative care for patients with metastatic non-small-cell lung cancer. N Engl J Med 2010;363(1):733–7422010.
4. Hannon B, Swami N, Rodin G, et al. Experiences of patients and caregivers with early palliative care: a qualitative study. Palliat Med 2017;31(1):72–81.
5. van Walree IC, Scheepers E, van Huis-Tanja L, et al. A systematic review on the association of the G8 with geriatric assessment, prognosis and course of treatment in older patients with cancer. J Geriatr Oncol 2019;10(6):847–58.
6. Ethun CG, Mehmet B, Jani AB, et al. Frailty and cancer: implications for oncology surgery, medical oncology, and radiation oncology. CA Cancer J Clin 2017;67(1): 363–77.
7. National Consensus Project for Quality Palliative Care Task Force. Clinical Practice Guidelines for Quality Palliative Care. 3rd ed. National Consensus Project for Quality Palliative Care; 2013.
8. Wildiers H, Heeren P, Puts M, et al. International Society of Geriatric Oncology consensus on geriatric assessment in older patients with cancer. J Clin Oncol 2014;32(24):2595–603.
9. Li D, Sun C, Kim H, et al. Geriatric Assessment–Driven Intervention (GAIN) on chemotherapy-related toxic effects in older adults with cancer: a randomized clinical trial. JAMA Oncol 2021;7(11). https://doi.org/10.1001/jamaoncol.2021.4158.
10. Burgess J, Ferdousi M, Gosal D, et al. Chemotherapy-induced peripheral neuropathy: epidemiology, pathomechanisms and treatment. Oncol Ther 2021;9(2): 385–450.
11. Gewandter JS, Fan L, Magnuson A, et al. Falls and functional impairments in cancer survivors with chemotherapy-induced peripheral neuropathy (CIPN): a University of Rochester CCOP study. Support Care Cancer 2013;21(7):2059–66.
12. Hesketh PJ, Kris MG, Basch E, et al. Antiemetics: ASCO guideline update. J Clin Oncol 2020;38(24):2782–97.

13. Balducci L. Geriatric oncology, spirituality, and palliative care. J Pain Symptom Manage 2019;57(1):171–5.
14. Developed by the American Geriatrics Society Ethnogeriatrics Committee. Achieving high-quality multicultural geriatric care. J Am Geriatr Soc 2016;64(2): 255–60.
15. Holman, C. (2019). Beers criteria updates: new guidance for geriatric medication safety. Wolters Kluwer. Available at: https://www.wolterskluwer.com/en/expert-insights/beers-criteria-updates-new-guidance-for-geriatric-medication-safety. Accessed May 4, 2023.
16. Sedrak MS, Freedman RA, Cohen HJ, et al. Older adult participation in cancer clinical trials: a systematic review of barriers and interventions. CA Cancer J Clin 2021;71(1):78–92.

Symptom Management in the Older Adult: 2023 Update

Augustin Joseph, MD[a],*, Balakrishna Vemula, MD[a,b],
Thomas J. Smith, MD[a,c]

KEYWORDS

- Constipation • Frailty • Geriatric • Depression • Nausea • Opioid • Pain • Palliative

KEY POINTS

- In the older adult with a serious illness, the goal of palliative medicine and symptom management is to optimize quality of life.
- There is a paucity of high-quality research in symptom management. Interventions should be individualized to each patient.
- Classify the correct type of pain: nociceptive versus neuropathic versus nociplastic.
- Patients and providers continue to have a general sense of fear and reluctance toward opioids.
- Non-pharmacologic interventions should be offered to all patients and can be useful in treatment of pain, fatigue, insomnia, and increase overall well-being.

INTRODUCTION

In the older adult with a serious illness, the goal of palliative medicine, especially when focusing on symptom management, is to optimize quality of life. As we discuss pain, constipation, fatigue, and other individual symptoms, it is paramount that we focus on the whole person. We must ask how our therapeutics is improving on quality-of-life measures such as independence, community building, and self-fulfillment more than the individual improvement of one symptom.

Frailty has become an overarching finding in many older adults with serious illness. Regardless of the serious illness (eg, cancer, heart failure, chronic obstructive pulmonary disease [COPD], dementia, and so forth), our patient should be assessed,

[a] Department of Medicine, Johns Hopkins Medical Institutions, 600 North Wolfe Street, Blalock 359, Baltimore, MD 21287, USA; [b] Department of Emergency Medicine, Johns Hopkins Medical Institutions, 600 North Wolfe Street, Blalock 359, Baltimore, MD 21287, USA; [c] Department of Oncology, Johns Hopkins Medical Institutions, 600 North Wolfe Street, Blalock 359, Baltimore, MD 21287, USA
* Corresponding author. 600 North Wolfe Street, Blalock 359, Baltimore, MD 21287, USA
E-mail address: ajosep30@jhmi.edu

Clin Geriatr Med 39 (2023) 449–463
https://doi.org/10.1016/j.cger.2023.04.006
0749-0690/23/© 2023 Elsevier Inc. All rights reserved.

geriatric.theclinics.com

reassessed, and managed according to their level of frailty. Symptom management options need to be considered in the lens of increasing frailty along an illness trajectory.

Since our last update in 2015, this field continues to be influenced by the opioid epidemic and the COVID-19 pandemic. Many of the general principles discussed in our previous iterations of this article in 2004 and 2015 have not changed, and a full review of individual symptoms is beyond the scope of this update.[1,2] Here, we will emphasize literature updates and best practices for the most common symptoms.

PAIN
Initial Considerations

Pain management in the older adult with a serious illness should focus on trusting our patient's pain experience and creating a therapeutic alliance focused on function and quality of life. The myth that pain is an expected part of aging continues to be a barrier in adequate reporting and optimal treatment.[3] Pain is still the predominant symptom that leads patients to access medical care.[4] Among older adults, chronic pain is common and can significantly diminish a person's quality of life.[5]

Patients may not be as forthcoming as we expect when reporting their pain level.[6] Misconceptions continue that pain is an expected part of aging leading to underreporting.[3] In addition, as we age a person's interpretation of pain can present as discomfort, aching, fatigue, and various other nonspecific symptoms.[7] The assessment of pain in individuals with neurocognitive disease presents as a significant barrier to optimal pain management as pain can present as delirium, restlessness, or agitation, which may lead to missing pain as the underlying cause of the distress.[8] Once pain is properly identified, many patients hesitate to add medications with concern for intolerable side effects such as somnolence and constipation.[9] There is also an overwhelming fear toward taking opioid pain medications with patients citing worry over the addiction potential even when they have low risk for addiction.[10]

Many of these fears stem from the opioid epidemic which continues to escalate.[11] Rates of overdose deaths involving prescription opioids are on the rise.[12] Older adults have the highest rates of being prescribed opioids compared with any other age group.[13] The level of opioid misuse in older adults needs to be further studied, as this population is at higher risk for complications from opioids.[14]

Pain Assessment

There are similar rates of acute pain among different age groups, whereas the prevalence of chronic pain (ie, pain lasting more than 3 months) increases as we age to the seventh decade and plateaus afterward.[5] Pain perception, intensity, and endurance change as we age, especially with a decrease in functionality of the body's pain inhibition systems.[15] It is now better understood that as we become older our pain threshold increases and our pain tolerance decreases.[16] In the older adult, a pain stimulus takes longer to be experienced as painful and is perceived as more intense.[17]

These data call into question the generalizability of the pain scales used in the adult population.[18] Recognizing and measuring pain in the older adult is challenging. Popular scales include numeric pain intensity scale, verbal descriptor scale, visual analog scale, Iowa pain thermometer, and the functional pain scale.[19] There are numerous studies comparing these scales, and there is no consensus for which scale is most reliable. The patient's self-report of pain continues to be the gold standard by which we should measure pain.[5]

Classifying the correct type of pain is essential and a basic outline is provided in **Table 1**.[1] Classically, pain has been classified as nociceptive, "pain that arises from

Table 1 Types of pain			
Types of pain	Nociceptive	Neuropathic	Nociplastic
Mechanism	Arises from actual or threatened damage to nonneural tissue and is due to the activation of nociceptors	Caused by a lesion or disease of the somatosensory nervous system	Arises from altered nociception despite no clear evidence of actual or threatened tissue damage causing the activation of peripheral nociceptors or evidence for disease or lesion of the somatosensory system causing the pain
Descriptors	Sharp, stabbing, dull, achy	Numbness, tingling, electric, allodynia	Widespread pain, hyperalgesia, allodynia, fatigue
Examples	Inflammatory/ischemic pain, mechanical injury, degenerative joint disease, cancer-related pain	Diabetic neuropathy, postherpetic neuralgia, chemotherapy-induced peripheral neuropathy, poststroke/spinal cord injury neuropathy	Irritable bowel syndrome, chronic pancreatitis, chronic pelvic pain, fibromyalgia
Treatment considerations	Physical interventions (yoga, tai chi, exercise), Psychological interventions (cognitive behavioral therapy, mindfulness, meditation)		
	NSAIDs; acetaminophen; steroids, opioids	Gabapentin, SNRIs; for severe cases consider opioids	Limited evidence/efficacy with pharmacologic agents; consider a trial of centrally acting agents such as SNRIs

Data from International Association for the Study of Pain.[20]

actual or threatened damage to non-neural tissue and is due to the activation of nociceptors," and neuropathic, "pain caused by a lesion or disease of the somatosensory nervous system."[20] In 2017, the International Association for the Study of Pain added a third category of nociplastic pain, "pain that arises from altered nociception despite no clear evidence of actual or threatened tissue damage causing the activation of peripheral nociceptors or evidence for disease or lesion of the somatosensory system causing the pain."[21] The mechanism of nociplastic pain is not fully understood. The pathophysiology is different from nociceptive and neuropathic pain and sometimes referred to as central sensitization. The underlying mechanism is thought to involve central nervous system changes to pain and sensory processing and can present with other central nervous system (CNS) symptoms such as fatigue, insomnia, and mood changes. For the older adult with a chronic serious illness, distinguishing nociplastic pain should be an important consideration because peripherally directed treatment strategies usually used for nociceptive or neuropathic pain may not be as effective.[22]

Pain and Frailty

After classifying the type of pain and before discussing treatment strategies, we must consider the narrow therapeutic window when aiming for optimal pain management in a frail person.[23] Polypharmacy is a major contributing factor to frailty, and a medication review with the goal of deprescribing should be our first step.[24] For instance, in patients with less than an estimated 2 years to live, statins can be safely discontinued and lead to a better quality of life.[25]

It is also important to establish measures of success and treatment goals with our patients before discussing management options. Many patients may say that their overall goal is to "have less pain," and we should encourage our patients to describe what having less pain will look like in their day-to-day life, and what functions they want to improve. In conjunction with the goal of decreasing pain, we should use this as an opportunity to establish tangible quality of life measures that can help evaluate the effectiveness of the chosen treatment overall. The intervention for improving pain should in some way also increase the patient's function/independence, access to resources, and/or community engagement.[26]

Pain Management with Adjuvant Agents

Non-pharmacologic techniques should be considered and offered to all patients. These interventions can be divided into physical and psychological interventions and are expanded on in **Table 2**.[27] There are numerous topical medications that can be used independently or in conjunction with systemic options reviewed in **Table 3**.

Acetaminophen is used as the first-line agent for the treatment of mild to moderate pain. It is well tolerated, inexpensive, and easy to access. Maximum daily dose of acetaminophen has come under contention. Historically, this was 4000 mg, and now maximum recommended daily dose of acetaminophen is 3000 mg.[28] However, in those who are frail, 80 years or older and have significant organ dysfunction or at risk of hepatoxicity, a maximum of 2000 mg is suggested.[28] Even when patients have liver failure, up to 2000 mg a day seems to be safe.

Non-steroidal anti-inflammatory drugs (NSAIDs) can be highly effective for mild to moderate pain with anti-inflammatory and analgesic properties.[29] Providers should monitor for side effects including gastrointestinal toxicities, cardiovascular adverse effects, and nephrotoxicity.[30] These toxicities are more commonly seen with higher cumulative doses, so for acute pain an NSAID may be reasonable for a short duration.[31]

Muscle relaxants such as cyclobenzaprine, baclofen, and methocarbamol should be avoided in the older adult.

Glucocorticoids for pain have a general lack of evidence base.[32] However, they are sometimes effective in clinical practice for patients especially in cancer pain with bone metastases, malignant bowel obstruction, headache caused by increased intracranial pressure, or organ capsular stretch from space occupying lesion. Glucocorticoids can also be used as an adjuvant agent during a pain crisis in patients who are not responding to escalating opioids.

Locally injected analgesia including joint injections and trigger point injections may be effective when trying to avoid systemic therapy. However, analgesic efficacy can wean over time. In patients with osteoarthritis, injections every 3 months can worsen cartilage damage.[33]

Pain Management with Neuropathic Agents

Neuropathic pain can be a result of peripheral nerve injury (eg, diabetic neuropathy, postherpetic neuralgia, chemotherapy-induced neuropathy) or central nerve

Table 2		
Examples of non-pharmacologic interventions for pain		
Method	**Indication**	**Comments**
Physical/Stimulatory		
Rehabilitation Physical therapy, therapeutic exercise	Musculoskeletal pain, deconditioning	Consider for all patients needing to meet functional goals
Mind/body Yoga, tai chi	Certain cancer-related pain, osteoarthritis, fibromyalgia	Many resources available online
Complementary Acupuncture, acupressure, reflexology	Pain related to cancer treatment, chronic pain	Several access issues including availability of providers and significant cost
Physiologic		
Behavioral therapy Cognitive behavioral therapy, biofeedback	Mixed pain, nociplastic pain	Consider for all patient with concurrent psychologic needs
Distraction Guided imagery, virtual reality, music therapy, deep breathing	Acute or chronic pain	Many resources available online
Integrative/Emerging		
Comprehensive pain programs	Mixed pain with significant loss of physical and mental abilities to function	Limited by availability of programs and variations between each make it difficult to generalize between programs
Scrambler Therapy	Neuropathic pain, nociplastic pain	>50% pain relief within days and lasting months; cost and access to providers are barrier

Data from 2015 Update[1] and The Consortium Pain Task Force White Paper.[27]

injury (eg, central poststroke pain syndrome, multiple sclerosis, spinal cord injury).[34] Gabapentinoids, such as gabapentin and pregabalin, and noradrenergic antidepressants, such as serotonin-norepinephrine reuptake inhibitors, are the first-line agents for neuropathic pain and can also be effective for nociplastic pain.[35] It is also effective for arthritis pain with manageable side effects.[36] Tricyclic antidepressants (ie, amitriptyline and nortriptyline) also have noradrenergic properties, but they are generally not used in the older adult given higher side effect profile compared with gabapentinoids and serotonin and norepinephrine reuptake inhibitors (SNRIs).

Providers should make a shared decision with the patient after discussing the risks/benefits between a gabapentinoid and SNRI. For example, in patients with kidney disease, gabapentin will require dose adjustment. Also, SNRIs should be avoided in patients with liver dysfunction. In patients who have concurrent depression or would prefer a once daily medication, an SNRI may be the preferred option. Relief from neuropathic pain with these medications is not instantaneous, and patients should trial the medication for at least 4 to 6 weeks. If there are no changes in pain after this period, it would be reasonable to switch to another agent.

Table 3
Topical pain medications

Agent	Comments
Menthol, camphor, and methyl salicylate	Various combinations, concentrations, and formulations are readily available over the counter and well tolerated
Topical NSAIDs	Such as diclofenac Use for musculoskeletal and osteoarthritic pain Minimal systemic absorption so can be an option in a patient who otherwise would not be a candidate for systemic NSAID therapy
Capsaicin	Selectively activates transient receptor potential vanilloid 1 (TRPV1) Can be used to treat neuropathic and osteoarthritic pain Low concentration formulations are readily available over the counter High concentration patches (8%) can be beneficial in postherpetic neuralgia, HIV-neuropathy, and diabetic neuropathy in individuals who are able to tolerate high concentration capsaicin which must be administered in a medical setting often needing pretreatment with local anesthetic
Lidocaine/prilocaine	Effective for localized superficial pain Various formulations are available Lidocaine/prilocaine cream has been shown to be effective for patients with painful wounds, ulcers, or hemorrhoids Used for diabetic peripheral neuropathy, chronic lower back pain, carpal tunnel syndrome, and osteoarthritis

Data from Lexicomp Online.

Pain Management with Opioids

Opioids are effective pain medications. As in 2002 and in 2015: "opioids remain the cornerstone of pain management." When prescribing opioids in the older adult, we must consider.

- There is a general sense of fear toward opioids in the public. Many patients are reluctant to an opioid trial, and some providers refuse to prescribe opioids.
- Once the decision is made to start an opioid, start at the lowest possible dose.
- The terminology we use for opioids (eg, immediate/sustained/extended-release vs short/long acting) can be very confusing to the lay person. Patient and family education on opioids should be highlighted on initiation and all follow-up visits.
- All patients should be educated that "immediate release" oral opioids can take up to an hour to reach its full effect and typically last 3 to 4 hours.
- If a patient is needing several doses of immediate release opioid over 24 hours or having to wake up at night to take additional doses, consider adding a sustained release opioid.
- Patients should only be on one immediate release opioid and one sustained release opioid.
- Patients on a sustained release opioid should have an immediate release opioid available for breakthrough pain at about 10% of their sustained release daily dose.
- Patients should be encouraged to keep an opioid administration log. There are several apps available for smart phones which can greatly help in this process for the technologically savvy older adult.
- Prescribe naloxone and a bowel regimen to all patients.

When choosing an opioid, have a conversation with your patient on what has worked for them in the past. For pain related to a serious illness, initiation of morphine, oxycodone, or hydromorphone is usually preferred over opioids that are compounded with acetaminophen or an NSAID. The decision among morphine, oxycodone, or hydromorphone should be based on your patient's characteristics, but most of the time the decision is driven by which opioid their insurance company will cover. Sustained-release opioids generally require a prior authorization and present a significant barrier to patient access. Many pharmacies carry a limited supply of sustained-release opioids. Opioid conversion tables offer basic guidelines when switching between opioid classes and oral/transdermal/parenteral formulations. Variations in absorption, metabolism, and excretion need to be considered for the individual patient especially in the geriatric setting. The terminology of "oral morphine equivalents" gives a false sense of equality when converting between opioids and a more apt term would be "oral morphine approximations."

Tramadol has fallen out of favor given its unpredictable metabolism. Tramadol is structurally an SNRI that is metabolized into an opioid, O-desmethyltramadol, by CYP2D6. Historically, many providers used tramadol as a step below starting a full opioid. It is now generally accepted to avoid tramadol completely and prescribe an opioid.[37] Buprenorphine opioid receptor agonist/antagonist is emerging as an opioid of choice for older adults. It has better safety profile than other opioids and does not have to be adjusted for renal insufficiency. Its transdermal preparation of 5 mcg/h is a long-acting preparation that can be started safety in an opioid naive patient, which may be of benefit for patients who are nonverbal and have severe cognitive impair who require opioid pain control.[38,39]

FATIGUE

Fatigue is the most common symptom described in older adults. Between 40% and 70% of older adults with chronic disease report fatigue, and greater than 75% of patients over the age of 70 years report fatigue on hospital admission.[40] The prevalence of fatigue in patients continues to increase with serious illness at end of life.[41] Early interventions are the key when considering treatment of fatigue in the older adult as fatigue increases the risk of negative health outcomes.[42]

Our first step in management should be identifying and treating reversible causes of fatigue. If reversible causes are not found, options for the treatment of fatigue are limited. The evidence base for these interventions is lacking because of limited studies, so the decision to trial an intervention should be individualized to your patient. Several options are discussed in **Box 1**.[43–50]

NEUROLOGIC AND PSYCHIATRIC SYMPTOMS
Depression/Anxiety

The prevalence of major depressive disorder has been rising in the older adult.[51] Risk factors for depression increase as we age and contribute to neurobiological/chemical changes.[52] The connection between depression and increased frailty is well established, each being a risk factor for the other.[53] We recommend all older patients with a serious illness should be screened for depression with the Patient Health Questionnaire 2 (PHQ-2) on a regular basis. Management of depression should be individualized; however, most effective interventions include both pharmacotherapy and psychotherapy. Clinical practice guidelines and treatments tailored toward the older adult should be emphasized. For example, SNRIs are associated with a greater occurrence of adverse events including falls in the older adult compared with SSRIs.[54] On the other

---

Box 1
Interventions for fatigue

Non-pharmacologic interventions:
- Exercise rehabilitation should be considered if the patient is able to tolerate it.
- Yoga and tai chi have a considerable evidence base in the treatment of cancer-related fatigue. Access to resources has been increasing and there are many self-guided videos that can be offered to patients.
- Sleep optimization through specific cognitive behavioral therapy for insomnia (CBT-I) has been shown to be effective.
- Nutrition should be evaluated and a referral to a dietician or speech therapy should be considered for select patients.

Pharmacologic interventions
- Glucocorticoids can improve fatigue in patients with serious illnesses included advanced cancer. Dexamethasone is most well studied with several randomized control trials. Long-term use of these medications should be cautioned given its side effect profile.
- Megestrol has fallen out of favor given significant side effect profile and potential increase in mortality.
- Psychostimulants have a limited role in the treatment of fatigue but may be beneficial to patients on a case-by-case basis. Methylphenidate has data from uncontrolled trial for patients with breast cancer and exceedingly high levels of fatigue. Modafinil has data in patients with Parkinson disease and obstructive sleep apnea.
- American ginseng has been shown in some studies to improve fatigue and should be used with caution given potential drug interactions.

Data from Refs.[42–49]

---

hand, if the patient has concurrent neuropathic pain or chronic low back pain, an SNRI may be a better option. In addition, psychotherapy interventions such as life review and dignity therapy should be offered especially when trying to minimize pill burden.[55,56]

Insomnia

Sleep patterns change as we age, and insomnia can greatly diminish quality of life. Cognitive behavioral therapy for insomnia (CBT-I) has been shown to be highly effective and should be used as our first-line intervention.[46] The basic principles of CBT-I can be discussed with patients in the office. A referral to a CBT-I specialist can be helpful for patients who have continued insomnia. CBT-I was found to have sustained reduction in insomnia months after intervention and may have overlapping benefit in improvement of pain in patients with osteoarthritis.[57] Use sedative hypnotics with caution secondary to risk of falls, delirium, and drug interaction. Ramelteon is a melatonin 1/2 receptor agonist with rapid absorption and has shown to reduce sleep latency. It has a low side effect profile and shows no evidence to data for rebound insomnia.[58]

Delirium

The general principles in the diagnosis and management of delirium have not changed. An acute change with waxing and waning consciousness, cognition, and attention should make us suspect delirium. First, we should address reversible causes, rule out infection, and review the patient's medications. Distinction should be made between hyperactive and hypoactive delirium, with the latter being less recognized.[59] There is almost a three-fold incremental risk for delirium in the frail patient.[60] Prevention is the key. A 2021 Cochrane review for the prevention of delirium cited moderate certainty evidence that nonpharmacologic interventions can reduce delirium incidence by 43% compared with usual care.[61] Early mobilization and sleep hygiene are the key components of these non-pharmacologic interventions. The neuropsychiatric side effects of steroids can usually be entirely mitigated by a small dose of olanzapine, 2.5 mg/h.[62]

RESPIRATORY SYMPTOMS
Dyspnea

Dyspnea is the subjective uncomfortable feeling of breathlessness. This sensation can be present independent of if the patient is experiencing hypoxia. The optimal first step to treat dyspnea, as is with many other symptoms, is to address the underlying etiology. For example, in the setting of COPD or asthma with wheezing, inhaled albuterol or ipratropium may be the solution. Bilevel ventilation may also provide relief. For someone with congestive heart failure (CHF) and volume overload, gentle diuresis may improve symptoms.

For symptoms that are present despite treating the underlying etiology, there are several options.[63] If the patient is hypoxic, then supplemental oxygen can likely help dyspnea. If the patient is dyspneic, but not hypoxic, then either supplemental oxygen or a bedside fan may be used. A 2020 systematic review published in JAMA Oncology assessed three studies specifically using fan-to-face therapy versus sham, and it showed that fan-to-face therapy is effective in relieving breathlessness. There is some evidence suggesting integrative medicine techniques, such as acupressure and reflexology, may be helpful in relieving dyspnea. Not surprisingly, when combining several different interventions, such as rehabilitation, behavioral and psychosocial education, and integrative medicine, there was also some improvement in dyspnea.[64]

Opioids are often the go-to medication to treat dyspnea in patients with serious illness.[63]

Low-dose short-acting opioids dosed every 4 to 6 hours are traditionally used for dyspnea. Recently, there has been some uncertainty regarding the effectiveness of long-acting formulations and their ability to relieve dyspnea. Two 2022 randomized controlled trials of low-dose extended-release morphine in patients with COPD experiencing chronic breathlessness showed no significant reduction in the intensity of breathlessness.[65,66] More evidence is needed to determine if this study can be extrapolated to other patient populations.

Dyspnea can trigger a cycle of anxiety and panic. One option to break this cycle is using benzodiazepines.[63] Non-pharmacologic adjuncts, such as deep breathing and sequential muscle relaxation techniques, are also particularly helpful in breaking the cycle.[64]

Cough

Coughing is a natural response to clear the airway. If it is persistent, then cough suppressants are an option. If dyspnea is concurrent with cough, a low-dose opioid as discussed earlier may be indicated. Over-the-counter agents such as dextromethorphan and anesthetizing throat lozenges may also provide relief. If associated with congestion, patients may benefit from hydration and guaifenesin. Gabapentin has been shown in a randomized trial to reduce coughing substantially and is routinely used in cancer and non-cancer patients by pulmonologists.[67,68] Nebulized hypertonic saline may facilitate clearing thicker secretions. If chronic and persistent, patients may benefit from a trial of gabapentin.[67]

GASTROINTESTINAL SYMPTOMS
Constipation

As is often the case with other symptoms, accurate diagnosis and etiology are crucial in both prevention and treatment. It is important to exclude alternative diagnoses, such as bowel obstruction, which may require surgical intervention. If fecal impaction is present, then manual disimpaction is required before medications. When treating constipation, there are both non-pharmacologic and pharmacologic approaches and often both are used simultaneously. Non-pharmacologic approaches include staying well hydrated, increasing dietary fiber intake, and increasing daily activity.

There are several classes of medications available to treat constipation.

- Bulk-forming agents such as psyllium fiber supplements are available over the counter. It requires the patient to be well hydrated; otherwise, it could worsen constipation.
- Osmotic agents also require the patient to be hydrated as they pull water into the intestinal lumen.
  - Polyethylene glycol is a commonly used over-the-counter agent. The starting dose is 17 g mixed into 8 ounces of liquid. This may not be ideal for patients with limited oral intake or volume-sensitive patients, such as those with renal impairment or CHF.
  - Lactulose or magnesium citrate, especially in volume-sensitive patients, is an effective alternative because it is a small volume per dose. The downside is that it is often accompanied by abdominal cramping and flatulence.
- Stimulants are a class of medications that can be used both daily and as a rescue medication.
  - Senna is often used daily to prevent constipation. The tablets are commonly used and have a wide dose range that can be titrated to effect—for some patients this is one bowel movement a day or every other day.
  - Bisacodyl is an effective stimulant that has both oral and rectal suppository formulations. The suppository is often used as a rescue medication when a patient has not had a bowel movement in 72 hours.
- Peripheral opioid reversal may be indicated if opioid-induced constipation is suspected, and it is refractory to other treatments.
  - Methylnaltrexone is an example of this class of medication. Caution should be used when prescribing this as it can cause abdominal cramping and in the presence of a bowel obstruction, potentially bowel perforation.
- Enemas are a good option if oral medications have not yielded results. Several distinct types of enemas are available. Caution should be used when selecting an enema based on the patient's medical history. In general, tap water or soap suds enemas are a safe choice.
- A note about docusate—A 2013 randomized, double-blind, placebo-controlled trial assessing docusate in the management of constipation showed no difference between docusate and placebo in treating constipation.[69]

Nausea and Vomiting

The differential for nausea and vomiting is broad. Identifying the trigger can help optimize treatment. Wood and colleagues summarizes four major centers that can trigger nausea—cortical, vestibular, chemoreceptor/toxin, and gastrointestinal.[70]

- A first-line agent that most individuals reach for is ondansetron or metoclopramide.
- If bowel edema or elevated intracranial pressure is the suspected etiology, then dexamethasone may provide relief.
- If the patient is experiencing dizziness, then anticholinergics may provide relief as they target the vestibular center.
- If a metabolic derangement or toxin is suspected, then an antidopaminergic agent could be used. Avoid antidopaminergic agents in patients with known or suspected Parkinson disease.

- Olanzapine has activity on several chemoreceptors involved in nausea and vomiting and has been shown to be highly effective for cancer-related nausea and may be effective for nausea/vomiting from other causes.[71,72] If the goals are to avoid pills, low-dose olanzapine at nighttime may be effective.

Cachexia/Anorexia

Unfortunately, there are no currently available medications that can directly reverse cachexia and anorexia from a serious illness. The best strategy is to treat any underlying etiology. For cancer anorexia cachexia syndrome (CACS), high protein and calorie foods and drinks have not been shown to cause weight gain even if patients have limited daily oral intake. We suspect alterations in neurohormonal balance as the root cause of CACS. In patients with advanced dementia, it is not recommended to pursue artificial nutrition.

MISCELLANEOUS BOTHERSOME SYMPTOMS

Itching: Initial therapies include topical cooling agents and antihistamines. Gabapentin may be effective for itching related to uremia, neuropathic pruritus, histamine release, and idiopathic/generalized pruritus. Methylnaltrexone can be considered for itching related to liver disease, bile cholestasis, and opioid-induced pruritus.

Hiccups: Persistent hiccups require a workup. Empiric treatment with a proton pump inhibitor (PPI) should be considered if gastroesophageal reflux disease (GERD) is suspected. Other agents to consider include baclofen or gabapentin.[73]

SUMMARY

Individualize symptom management for the older adult with a serious illness by focusing on quality of life. There is a general lack of research in this field. Non-pharmacologic interventions should be offered to all patients and can be useful in treatment of pain, fatigue, insomnia, and increase overall well-being. Pain management starts with trusting your patient's pain experience narrative and focusing on their functional goals.

CLINICS CARE POINTS

- In the older adult with a serious illness, the goal of palliative medicine and symptom management is to optimize quality of life.
- There is a paucity of high-quality research in symptom management. Interventions should be individualized to each patient.
- Classify the correct type of pain: nociceptive versus neuropathic versus nociplastic.
- Patients and providers continue to have a general sense of fear and reluctance toward opioids.
- Non-pharmacologic interventions should be offered to all patients and can be useful in treatment of pain, fatigue, insomnia, and increase overall well-being.

ACKNOWLEDGMENTS

Julie M Waldfogel, Pharm D, for contributions to the fatigue and neurological/psychiatric symptoms sections.

DISCLOSURE

The authors have nothing to disclose.

REFERENCES

1. Smith TJ. Symptom management in the older adult: 2015 update. Clin Geriatr Med 2015;31(2):155–75.
2. Brown JA, Von Roenn JH. Symptom management in the older adult. Clin Geriatr Med 2004;20(4):621–40, v–vi.
3. Thielke S, Sale J, Reid MC. Aging: are these 4 pain myths complicating care? J Fam Pract 2012;61(11):666–70.
4. Yong RJ, Mullins PM, Bhattacharyya N. Prevalence of chronic pain among adults in the United States. Pain 2022;163(2):e328.
5. Bicket MC, Mao J. Chronic pain in older adults. Anesthesiol Clin 2015;33(3):577–90.
6. Levy AG, Scherer AM, Zikmund-Fisher BJ, et al. Prevalence of and factors associated with patient nondisclosure of medically relevant information to clinicians. JAMA Netw Open 2018;1(7):e185293.
7. Mun S, Park K, Baek Y, et al. Interrelationships among common symptoms in the elderly and their effects on health-related quality of life: a cross-sectional study in rural Korea. Health Qual Life Outcome 2016;14(1):146.
8. Hadjistavropoulos T, Herr K, Prkachin KM, et al. Pain assessment in elderly adults with dementia. Lancet Neurol 2014;13(12):1216–27.
9. Wang Y, Li X, Jia D, et al. Exploring polypharmacy burden among elderly patients with chronic diseases in Chinese community: a cross-sectional study. BMC Geriatr 2021;21(1):308.
10. Page R, Blanchard E. Opioids and cancer pain: patients' needs and access challenges. JOP 2019;15(5):229–31.
11. Schepis TS, McCabe SE, Teter CJ. Sources of opioid medication for misuse in older adults: results from a nationally representative survey. Pain 2018;159(8):1543–9.
12. Abuse NI on D. Overdose Death Rates. National Institute on Drug Abuse. Published January 20, 2022. Available at: https://nida.nih.gov/research-topics/trends-statistics/overdose-death-rates. Accessed December 9, 2022.
13. Han B, Compton WM, Blanco C, et al. Prescription opioid use, misuse, and use disorders in U.S. Adults: 2015 national survey on drug use and health. Ann Intern Med 2017;167(5):293–301.
14. Maree RD, Marcum ZA, Saghafi E, et al. A systematic review of opioid and benzodiazepine misuse in older adults. Am J Geriatr Psychiatr 2016;24(11):949–63.
15. González-Roldán AM, Terrasa JL, Sitges C, et al. Age-related changes in pain perception are associated with altered functional connectivity during resting state. Front Aging Neurosci 2020;12. Available at: https://www.frontiersin.org/articles/10.3389/fnagi.2020.00116. Accessed December 21, 2022.
16. Lautenbacher S. Experimental approaches in the study of pain in the elderly. Pain Med 2012;13(Suppl 2):S44–50.
17. Lautenbacher S, Peters JH, Heesen M, et al. Age changes in pain perception: a systematic-review and meta-analysis of age effects on pain and tolerance thresholds. Neurosci Biobehav Rev 2017;75:104–13.
18. Schofield P, Abdulla A. Pain assessment in the older population: what the literature says. Age Ageing 2018;47(3):324–7.
19. Bullock L, Bedson J, Jordan JL, et al. Pain assessment and pain treatment for community-dwelling people with dementia: a systematic review and narrative synthesis. Int J Geriatr Psychiatry 2019;34(6):807–21.

20. Terminology | International Association for the Study of Pain. International Association for the Study of Pain (IASP). Available at: https://www.iasp-pain.org/resources/terminology/. Accessed December 21, 2022.

21. Nijs J, Lahousse A, Kapreli E, et al. Nociplastic pain criteria or recognition of central sensitization? Pain phenotyping in the past, present and future. J Clin Med 2021;10(15):3203.

22. Fitzcharles MA, Cohen SP, Clauw DJ, et al. Nociplastic pain: towards an understanding of prevalent pain conditions. Lancet 2021;397(10289):2098–110.

23. Tinnirello A, Mazzoleni S, Santi C. Chronic pain in the elderly: mechanisms and distinctive features. Biomolecules 2021;11(8):1256.

24. Ali A, Arif AW, Bhan C, et al. Managing chronic pain in the elderly: an overview of the recent therapeutic advancements. Cureus 2018;10(9):e3293.

25. Kutner JS, Blatchford PJ, Taylor DH, et al. Safety and benefit of discontinuing statin therapy in the setting of advanced, life-limiting illness. JAMA Intern Med 2015;175(5):691–700.

26. Function-Based Objectives | Treatment Planning. Pain Management. Available at: https://www.ihs.gov/painmanagement/treatmentplanning/functionbasedobjectives/. Accessed January 2, 2023.

27. Tick H, Nielsen A, Pelletier KR, et al. Evidence-based nonpharmacologic strategies for comprehensive pain care: the Consortium pain Task Force white paper. EXPLORE 2018;14(3):177–211.

28. Acetaminophen. Lexi-Drugs. Hudson, OH: Lexicomp, 2015. Available at: http://online.lexi.com/. Accessed January 2, 2023.

29. Malec M, Shega JW. Pain management in the elderly. Med Clin North Am 2015;99(2):337–50.

30. Wongrakpanich S, Wongrakpanich A, Melhado K, et al. A comprehensive review of non-steroidal anti-inflammatory drug use in the elderly. Aging Dis 2018;9(1):143–50.

31. Gooch K, Culleton BF, Manns BJ, et al. NSAID use and progression of chronic kidney disease. Am J Med 2007;120(3):280.e1–7.

32. Haywood A, Good P, Khan S, et al. Corticosteroids for the management of cancer-related pain in adults. Cochrane Database Syst Rev 2015;2015(4):CD010756.

33. McAlindon TE, LaValley MP, Harvey WF, et al. Effect of intra-articular triamcinolone vs saline on knee cartilage volume and pain in patients with knee osteoarthritis: a randomized clinical trial. JAMA 2017;317(19):1967–75.

34. Giovannini S, Coraci D, Brau F, et al. Neuropathic pain in the elderly. Diagnostics 2021;11(4):613.

35. Tauben D. Nonopioid medications for pain. Phys Med Rehabil Clin N Am 2015;26(2):219–48.

36. Du Z, Chen H, Cai Y, et al. Pharmacological use of gamma-aminobutyric acid derivatives in osteoarthritis pain management: a systematic review. BMC Rheumatol 2022;6(1):28.

37. Smith A. Tramadon't: a podcast with David Juurlink about the dangers of Tramadol. A Geriatrics and Palliative Care Podcast for Every Healthcare Professional. Published June 27, 2018. Available at: https://geripal.org/tramadont-dangers-of-tramadol/. Accessed January 2, 2023.

38. Kang C. Opioid misuse in older patients requires careful consideration of many factors. Drugs & Therapy Perspectives; 2022. p. 1–5.

39. Bissaillon A, Mesa S, Ana MD, et al. Is buprenorphine safe for the treatment of chronic pain in adults? Evidence-Based Practice 2022;25(9):18–9.

40. Torossian M, Jacelon CS. Chronic illness and fatigue in older individuals: a systematic review. Rehabil Nurs 2021;46(3):125–36.
41. Kutner JS, Kassner CT, Nowels DE. Symptom burden at the end of life: hospice providers' perceptions. J Pain Symptom Manage 2001;21(6):473–80.
42. Knoop V, Cloots B, Costenoble A, et al. Fatigue and the prediction of negative health outcomes: a systematic review with meta-analysis. Ageing Res Rev 2021;67:101261.
43. Pyszora A, Budzyński J, Wójcik A, et al. Physiotherapy programme reduces fatigue in patients with advanced cancer receiving palliative care: randomized controlled trial. Support Care Cancer 2017;25(9):2899–908.
44. Dong B, Xie C, Jing X, et al. Yoga has a solid effect on cancer-related fatigue in patients with breast cancer: a meta-analysis. Breast Cancer Res Treat 2019; 177(1):5–16.
45. Wayne PM, Lee MS, Novakowski J, et al. Tai Chi and Qigong for cancer-related symptoms and quality of life: a systematic review and meta-analysis. J Cancer Surviv 2018;12(2):256–67.
46. Qaseem A, Kansagara D, Forciea MA, et al. Clinical guidelines committee of the American college of physicians. Management of chronic insomnia disorder in adults: a clinical practice guideline from the American college of physicians. Ann Intern Med 2016;165(2):125–33.
47. Ruiz Garcia V, López-Briz E, Carbonell Sanchis R, et al. Megestrol acetate for treatment of anorexia-cachexia syndrome. Cochrane Database Syst Rev 2013; 2013(3):CD004310.
48. Yennurajalingam S, Palmer JL, Chacko R, et al. Factors associated with response to methylphenidate in advanced cancer patients. Oncol 2011;16(2):246–53.
49. Kuan YC, Wu D, Huang KW, et al. Effects of modafinil and armodafinil in patients with obstructive sleep apnea: a meta-analysis of randomized controlled trials. Clin Ther 2016;38(4):874–88.
50. Barton DL, Liu H, Dakhil SR, et al. Wisconsin Ginseng (Panax quinquefolius) to improve cancer-related fatigue: a randomized, double-blind trial, N07C2. J Natl Cancer Inst 2013;105(16):1230–8.
51. Abdoli N, Salari N, Darvishi N, et al. The global prevalence of major depressive disorder (MDD) among the elderly: a systematic review and meta-analysis. Neurosci Biobehav Rev 2022;132:1067–73.
52. Maier A, Riedel-Heller SG, Pabst A, et al. Risk factors and protective factors of depression in older people 65+. A systematic review. PLoS One 2021;16(5): e0251326.
53. Soysal P, Veronese N, Thompson T, et al. Relationship between depression and frailty in older adults: a systematic review and meta-analysis. Ageing Res Rev 2017;36:78–87.
54. Sobieraj DM, Martinez BK, Hernandez AV, et al. Adverse effects of pharmacologic treatments of major depression in older adults. J Am Geriatr Soc 2019; 67(8):1571–81.
55. Al-Ghafri BR, Al-Mahrezi A, Chan MF. Effectiveness of life review on depression among elderly: a systematic review and meta-analysis. Pan Afr Med J 2021; 40:168.
56. Kredentser MS, Chochinov HM. Psychotherapeutic considerations for patients with terminal illness. APT 2020;73(4):137–43.
57. Vitiello MV, Rybarczyk B, Von Korff M, et al. Cognitive behavioral therapy for insomnia improves sleep and decreases pain in older adults with Co-morbid insomnia and osteoarthritis. J Clin Sleep Med 2009;5(4):355–62.

58. Sateia MJ, Kirby-Long P, Taylor JL. Efficacy and clinical safety of ramelteon: an evidence-based review. Sleep Med Rev 2008;12(4):319–32.
59. van Velthuijsen EL, Zwakhalen SMG, Mulder WJ, et al. Detection and management of hyperactive and hypoactive delirium in older patients during hospitalization: a retrospective cohort study evaluating daily practice. Int J Geriatr Psychiatry 2018;33(11):1521–9.
60. Zhang XM, Jiao J, Xie XH, et al. The association between frailty and delirium among hospitalized patients: an updated meta-analysis. J Am Med Dir Assoc 2021;22(3):527–34.
61. Burton JK, Craig LE, Yong SQ, et al. Non-pharmacological interventions for preventing delirium in hospitalised non-ICU patients. Cochrane Database Syst Rev 2021;7(7):CD013307.
62. Akid I, Nesbit S, Nanavati J, et al. Prevention of steroid-induced neuropsychiatric complications with neuroleptic drugs: a review. Am J Hosp Palliat Care 2022; 39(4):472–6.
63. Feliciano JL, Waldfogel JM, Sharma R, et al. Pharmacologic interventions for breathlessness in patients with advanced cancer: a systematic review and meta-analysis. JAMA Netw Open 2021;4(2):e2037632.
64. Gupta A, Sedhom R, Sharma R, et al. Nonpharmacological interventions for managing breathlessness in patients with advanced cancer: a systematic review. JAMA Oncol 2021;7(2):290–8.
65. Ekström M, Ferreira D, Chang S, et al. Effect of regular, low-dose, extended-release morphine on chronic breathlessness in chronic obstructive pulmonary disease: the BEAMS randomized clinical trial. JAMA 2022;328(20):2022–32.
66. Verberkt CA, van den Beuken-van Everdingen MHJ, Schols JMGA, et al. Effect of sustained-release morphine for refractory breathlessness in chronic obstructive pulmonary disease on health status: a randomized clinical trial. JAMA Intern Med 2020;180(10):1306–14.
67. Ryan NM, Birring SS, Gibson PG. Gabapentin for refractory chronic cough: a randomised, double-blind, placebo-controlled trial. Lancet 2012;380(9853): 1583–9.
68. Razzak R, Waldfogel JM, Doberman DJ, et al. Gabapentin for cough in cancer. J Pain Palliat Care Pharmacother 2017;31(3–4):195–7.
69. Tarumi Y, Wilson MP, Szafran O, et al. Randomized, double-blind, placebo-controlled trial of oral docusate in the management of constipation in hospice patients. J Pain Symptom Manage 2013;45(1):2–13.
70. Wood GJ, Shega JW, Lynch B, et al. Management of intractable nausea and vomiting in patients at the end of life: "I was feeling nauseous all of the time . . . nothing was working. JAMA 2007;298(10):1196–207.
71. Navari RM, Pywell CM, Le-Rademacher JG, et al. Olanzapine for the treatment of advanced cancer-related chronic nausea and/or vomiting: a randomized pilot trial. JAMA Oncol 2020;6(6):895–9.
72. Davis MP, Sanger GJ. The benefits of olanzapine in palliating symptoms. Curr Treat Options Oncol 2020;22(1):5.
73. Steger M, Schneemann M, Fox M. Systemic review: the pathogenesis and pharmacological treatment of hiccups. Aliment Pharmacol Ther 2015;42(9):1037–50.

Global Geriatric Palliative Care

Nafiisah B.M.H. Rajabalee, MBBS[a],*, Augustin Joseph, MD[b],
Corey X. Tapper, MD, MS[b]

KEYWORDS

- Global public health • Global palliative care • Geriatrics • Frail seniors

KEY POINTS

- Global palliative care needs and access for seniors are largely unmet, especially for the underserved populations of the world.
- Existing successful care models of palliative care for seniors can be replicated with culturally appropriate adaptations.
- Education is the most powerful tool to identify and bridge gaps for geriatric palliative needs across societies.

INTRODUCTION

With increased life expectancy, the world population is aging.[1–3] Our seniors deserve quality care that is equitable to other age groups. Palliative medicine is increasingly recognized as a high value care service considering the holistic practice of medicine keeping the patient and care unit at the forefront. Many international organizations have paved the way to popularize palliative care across the globe, some visibly so, while others work arduously behind the scenes. The path to expand access to palliative care has come a long way. We look ahead, aware of challenges, and hopeful that with lessons learned from the past and continued innovation, we can pave the way for the future of geriatric palliative care.

PRESENT STATE

We live in a global village. International collaboration to tackle the world's healthcare challenges is of utmost value.[4] Although great strides have been achieved in medicine and in longevity in the last century, we remain cognizant that our skills and resources are suboptimally distributed. The world population is aging; in 2021, the World Data bank reported that around 10% of the 7.89 billion of the world's residents was aged

[a] Johns Hopkins School of Medicine, 600 North Wolfe Street, Blalock 359, Baltimore, MD 21287, USA; [b] Section of Palliative Medicine, Department of Medicine, Johns Hopkins Medical Institutions, 600 North Wolfe Street, Blalock 359, Baltimore, MD 21287, USA
* Corresponding author.
E-mail address: naf_rajabalee@yahoo.com

Clin Geriatr Med 39 (2023) 465–473
https://doi.org/10.1016/j.cger.2023.05.002
0749-0690/23/Published by Elsevier Inc.

older than 65 years. This demographic shift affects the state of global health. Chronological and biological age may differ by genetic and environmental influences.

Geriatric medicine focuses on the care of seniors, with promotion of preserved function, independence, quality of life, and prevention of institutionalization. Palliative medicine is a subspecialty focusing on quality of life with an interdisciplinary approach. The Center to Advance Palliative Care defines palliative care as "specialized medical care for people living with serious illness. This type of care is focused on providing relief from the symptoms and stress of the illness." It is traced back to the hospice movement in the United Kingdom in the 1950s. It is an added layer of support in expert symptom management, patient and "care unit" advocacy in decision-making, planning, and holistic support. Geriatric palliative medicine uses the principles from both subspecialties to best serve this age group.

Research in "geriatric palliative care" is in relatively early stages.[4] Data from the underserved populations of the world are lacking. Across the continents, progress varies across settings, with several countries well into expansion phases with geriatric palliative medicine part of their national health budgets.[5]

Very often, seniors are excluded from clinical trials. Despite this, the value of palliative care for the geriatric population is increasingly recognized. Palliative medicine indeed achieves the triple aims of the Institute for Healthcare Improvement: patient satisfaction, population health, and per capita cost.[6]

The second edition of the Global Atlas to Palliative Care highlights that "outside North America, Europe, and Australia, access to quality palliative care continues to be minimal even though 76% of the need is in low-and-middle-income countries." The panel estimates that 67% of the 20 million with palliative care needs at the end of life are more than 60 years old.[7]

Another study on the status of palliative care in 234 countries, areas or territories found that it was well integrated into healthcare systems in only 20 of them; 42% have no delivery system for palliative care services. In 32% of those countries, service delivery reaches only a small percentage of the population. Some 80% of the world's population lack adequate access to medication needed for palliative care.[8,9]

Advanced age is a risk factor for chronic diseases, malignancies, and geriatric syndromes (ie, frailty, vision, and hearing impairments, incontinence, and so forth). Often, seniors require functional status evaluation to offer the best management options that they can possibly tolerate. Best-case and worst-case scenarios take a different trajectory based on geriatric comorbidities and functional reserves. The Palliative Performance Scale is often used for the assessment of functional status.[10,11] Other indices within geriatrics include a comprehensive geriatric assessment or the G8 screening tool.[12]

The holistic approach of palliative medicine is aligned with goals of geriatric care to avoid overburdening patients while keeping in mind possible implicit biases of ageism. Patients may become overwhelmed by polypharmacy, desynchronized appointments with multiple subspecialties, and inaccurate medication reconciliations. Palliative care, by focusing on the goals and values of geriatric patients, can help avoid options patients deem burdensome while simultaneously respecting choices for treatment preferences. Being cognizant of these potential biases prepares us to better serve seniors with a person-centered approach. Part of age-friendly health care focuses on "What Matters Most" in order to offer value-concordant care.[13] It is imperative to discuss all options objectively.[14–16]

Early introduction of palliative care has been shown to reduce symptom and psychological burden for patients with advanced cancer and other serious illnesses. Patients who particularly benefit include those with heart failure,[17] chronic obstructive lung diseases,[18] amyotrophic lateral sclerosis,[19] human immunodeficiency virus,[20] and dementia.[21,22]

Palliative medicine providers specialize in communication skills; social and spiritual support; and symptom management such as delirium, moral distress, pain, dyspnea, nausea, vomiting, constipation, diarrhea, malignant bowel obstructions, depression and anxiety, and end of life symptom management.

Hospice is a service that delivers palliative care to patients and families at the end of life. Although policies in the United States require a prognosis of 6 months or less for hospice eligibility, other countries do not have such restrictions.[23] End-of-life can be a stressful time for patients, families, and clinicians. The Economist Intelligence Unit, a research department of the Economist group, developed a quality death index, based on the availability, cost, and quality of basic end-of-life healthcare. Their findings in 40 countries showed that affluent nations such as the United Kingdom, Australia, and New Zealand had better infrastructure and end-of-life care programs. Countries from Asia, Africa, and South America were rated as having poor death quality.[24] Lack of high-quality end-of-life care results in poor symptom management and preventable suffering. This is particularly so in pain management. Analgesia is a cornerstone of relieving suffering. The World Health Organization (WHO) named several essential medications, including opioids, as part of the human rights' obligations. Access remains a barrier, with low-income and middle-income countries accounting for only 10% of global opioid use.[7]

Geriatric palliative medicine is part of the answer to better managing our fragmented health systems for this age group. The Worldwide Hospice and Palliative Care Alliance, the International Palliative Care Initiative, the Center to Advance Palliative Care, and other similar organizations are championing pragmatic projects across communities. To support and scale improved access to geriatric palliative care for even more patients, every stratum of the community needs education. Palliative care needs of seniors can be added to curricula across the schools of healthcare providers, healthcare business, and administrative policy makers, who can in turn spread the knowledge. Support and advocacy from governments, academia, private organizations, and trans-sectoral leaders can catalyze the implementation of palliative care as a basic human right for the geriatric population.

There are several examples worldwide of successful models of care across different settings.[5,25–30] Whether it is integration into primary care, mobile clinics under a tree or at work places, community engagement plays a vital role in the deployment of care plans. There are many volunteers around the world making a difference, one community at a time.

In South Africa, projects funded by the Open Society Foundations' International Palliative Care Initiative have paved the way for palliative care programs across society with projects reaching correctional facilities.[31]

Another example of an impactful model of care is that at the Trivandrum Institute of Palliative Science in Kerala, pioneered by Dr M.R. Rajagopal, a Nobel Peace Prize Winner for his contribution to the relief of suffering in his community. India is home to more than 17% of the world's population. Some of the advocacy work he pioneered involved changing policies around availability of morphine, increasing awareness of palliative care by local communities, and filling the gap to access care through optimizing mentored volunteering and then monitoring the success through research. Indian undergraduate medical curricula now include palliative medicine. Furthermore, palliative care was integrated into primary care.

In yet another instance of expanding access to palliative care, Latin America's Pan American Health Organization built on the concept of Extension for Community

Healthcare Outcomes project. This is an educational tool developed by Dr Sanjeev Arora in Albuquerque, New Mexico, nearly 2 decades ago to tackle Hepatitis C. It is based on the motto "All Teach, All Learn" and maximizes finite specialist skills through videoconferencing, and mentoring front-liners and the community to bridge gaps in clinical care. This model has expanded across the world to Asia, Africa, and Europe for palliative medicine.

In October 2022, the World's Innovation Summit for Health in Doha, Qatar, published a report on integrating palliative care for older adults. This laudable collaboration involving the Worldwide Hospice and Palliative Care Organization, Alzheimer's Disease International and Lebanon's Hospice Association, based their recommendations of a needs' assessment tailored to the country. National strategies similar to the Indian project discussed above, incorporated all national stakeholders, policymakers, educationists, service providers, access to essential medicines, advocacy and awareness raising, and research in order to better support geriatric patients and their caregivers.[5]

In the sultanate of Oman, palliative care is nurse driven. Within this context, a collaboration with the oncology societies and nursing societies led to an initiative to include palliative care in nursing and other healthcare schools.[32] Countries in the region also participated in the training and took back skills to implement within their own communities.

Similar projects in several other countries are ongoing. With the recent developments in telemedicine, transcontinental collaboration is economically very feasible. It is time to further even more advocacy work and call to action organizations across the globe to join their efforts to create a worldwide symbiosis.[8] This would involve public and private stakeholders all unified under the vision of senior access to quality palliative care.

Resources, health, and technological literacy vary in healthcare systems around the world. Based on cultural norms and values across and within countries, patients may interpret and address suffering differently. However, there is a basic level of person-centered care that can be aimed for across cultures, which could lead to the development of universal standards for palliative delivery. However, there is a basic level of person-centered care that can be aimed for. The Lancet Commission on Palliative Care and Pain Relief aptly describes an "essential package of palliative care medicines, basic equipment and human resources to alleviate avoidable suffering in low- and middle-income countries."[33]

The need for palliative care for seniors is universal. With the growing aging population, it is imperative to train more providers in senior palliative care skills. To staff and develop palliative care specialist centers will take time. Specialist palliative care refers comes from providers who receive extensive clinical training in the field. This type of care is provided above and beyond the palliative care skills expected of a generalist.

In the interim, based on country-specific resources, existing volunteer healthcare organizations can receive training to provide basic-palliative or generalist-palliative services. Targeting interprofessional education centers with integrative palliative care and dialect-tailored communication skills can be a helpful strategy to encourage the next generation to take charge with burgeoning ideas within their specific contexts.

Outcome Measures

To track progress, objective measures of outcomes are essential. Medicine does not operate in isolation; it must draw on the expertise of policymakers, healthcare engineers, planners, and other specialists to develop effective strategic plans and organize cross-disciplinary services to develop global plans for palliative care delivery.

Of note, patient-centered care calls for the humanization of healthcare beyond metrics. Flourishing economics is a natural consequence of well-nurtured societies. It is hence primordial that our administrations and the corporate voice embrace the holistic approach of palliative care. Other barriers such as misconceptions and financial toxicity will need dismantling.

There are several individuals driving advancements in global palliative care. Dr Stoltenberg, a palliative care and global health specialist at Massachusetts General Hospital, is one such person. We had a brief discussion based on his work in the Caribbean and Latin America in countries such as Chile and Jamaica.[34]

A CONVERSATION WITH DR STOLTENBERG

Dr *Rajabalee*: What is the current state of geriatric global palliative care?

Dr *Stoltenberg*: We are at a unique point in the history of global palliative care, including the realm of geriatrics. For a very long time, it was a battle of convincing institutions and leaders around the world that it was important. Thanks to a lot of advocacy work, the Lancet Commission[30] being the most recent one, campaigns by the World Health Organization, the American Academy of Hospice and Palliative Medicine, the European Palliative Care association amongst others, palliative care has been brought to the forefront. We now have strong evidence-based ways in which palliative care improves healthcare outcomes and decreases costs when done well. We are now facing a new battle: It is about implementation- We all know the 'why' now. It is more about the 'how'. We are a few years into that and in its first few phases. However, most patients who need palliative care globally still do not have access to it. We now need to look at successful models and expand on them or replicate them.

Dr *Rajabalee*: What are we doing well?

Dr *Stoltenberg*: It is highly variable. Some regions are doing more effective work and expanding more rapidly than others. My experience is mostly in the Caribbean and Latin America including Chile, Columbia, and Jamaica. These regions are like many other parts of the world in the sense that they are incredibly heterogenous across and within countries. In Chile for example, in the urban areas, there is excellent access to basic palliative care services from outpatient to even home-based services for cancer patients. However, services are less robust in rural areas. There is also a huge variation in the quality of palliative care services from country to country. In some countries, Palliative care can be equated to pain management, and comprehensive interdisciplinary care beyond pain can be missing. However, pain management is a great place to start. India is very diverse. In Kerala, they integrated palliative care into primary care at a level rarely seen anywhere else in the world. However, there is still minimal palliative care services in many other parts of India.

Dr *Rajabalee*: What are some actionable points to overcome some barriers to geriatric palliative care?

Dr *Stoltenberg*: There are two strategies that are needed. First, it is important to partner with national and international groups-we do not need to re-invent the wheel. There are already a lot of high-quality education programs and strategies to create new programs and measure their impacts. There is no reason to start from scratch. At the same time, each time we build an integrated program, we need to culturally adapt it to the local setting; We need to respond to the ways in which patients suffer and utilize the unique cultural resources of healing and support. The core can be shared across cultures and settings. However, during integration, the cultural layer must be tailored and integrated.

Dr *Rajabalee*: What is your advice for the way forward?

Dr *Stoltenberg*: It is important to continue to invest in and support mentorship networks and relationships of palliative care leaders around the world. We can have regional hubs and international collaboration and partnership. Secondly, I think the current evidence base of palliative care too often comes from the West. We need an expansion of palliative care research and coming out of the global south so that the future of palliative care better reflects the diversity of suffering and healing around the world.

FUTURE DIRECTIONS

The work of Dr Stoltenberg and many others such as him highlight the need for improved access to palliative medicine around the world. This is especially important for older adults as our world population is living longer with chronic medical conditions. A one-size-fits-all model of palliative medicine is unlikely to work. Although there are universal common pathways in suffering and standards of care to alleviate them, it is important to consider cultural differences and values.

In order to account for these differences, proposed improved models for expanding palliative medicine resources should focus on.

1. Training/teaching the current and next generation of healthcare providers in communication, basic symptom management, and value-concordant care
2. Integrating palliative medicine into developing healthcare systems and
3. Access to essential medications for symptom management.

Training the current and future healthcare workforce in the principles of palliative care is of primary importance. Ground efforts, such as the ones implemented in Chile should be trialed at other universities through sponsorship and collaboration. Basic palliative principles such as serious illness communication, value-based shared decision-making, and symptom management need to be integrated into the curriculum of every healthcare trainee. Regional and International collaboration can lead to prolific progress. Telemedicine is a tool we can use for worldwide collaboration and partnerships.

Communication is a cornerstone of good healthcare and palliative care. Programs like VitalTalk and Serious Illness Conversation Guide have been effective measures in the United States to teach palliative medicine skills to nurses, medical students, pharmacists, and even medical professionals with many years of experience. The feasibility of translating and implanting these resources to areas of the world with limited resources to palliative medicine education needs further study.

When developing healthcare systems, integrating palliative care into primary care was an effective model in Kerala, India, as discussed earlier. This contrasts with how palliative care was established in developed nations such as the United States, in which it was added onto an already-developed healthcare system with varying levels of integration. In the United States and many other developed countries, ageing is treated as a medical problem—a trend, which is exemplified by record high institutionalization rates into nursing homes. It may be possible to reduce the medicalization of ageing by mirroring the efforts of organizations such as Pallium in Kerala, India, and integrating palliative medicine into primary and specialized care models such as geriatrics and oncology.

Systems also need to be developed to account for and mitigate suffering at the end of life. Access to symptom management medications, particularly opioids, continues to be limited in many parts of the world. Concerns like medication diversion will need elucidation and practical solutions. While developing healthcare systems for geriatric palliative care, there needs to be continued efforts and advocacy on a community and governmental level for better access to medications for symptom management such as pain, shortness of breath, nausea, constipation, and delirium.

SUMMARY

We have made great strides since Dame Cicely Saunders promulgated the palliative care movement. Despite unmet needs, increasing demands, and the potential for burnout, we are optimistic that international cooperation can improve access to palliative care for elderly individuals in low-income and middle-income countries and marginalized communities worldwide. The best route forward is a combination of community organization, international collaboration, government assistance, and education.

CLINICS CARE POINTS

- Telemedicine for long distance collaboration is a tool for global geriatric palliative care.
- Incorporating geriatric palliative care curricula in medical, nursing, public health, and clinical schools can train the next generation of healthcare providers in its basic tenets.
- Clarity about what palliative medicine is can help increase acceptance among patients and providers.
- We can tap into existing resources to act as screening agents or community educators-volunteers from nongovernmental organizations, religious communities to create culturally appropriate models of care.
- Quarterly regional symposia can follow-up on useful tactics and address challenges faced by patients and providers. Yearly international conferences can then assess if goals were met and for further refining of care models with room for adapting to specific country settings.
- National health budgets can have allocation for palliative medicine as a branch of population health.
- Pharmacists can become educators about WHO policies for appropriate use of medications including opioids.
- In some settings, medication diversion can become a barrier to care. Soliciting every layer of society to address this challenge is an ongoing effort.
- Ethical committees can be established as ombudsmen overseeing policy review.

ACKNOWLEDGMENTS

Mark Stoltenberg, MD, MA, Massachusetts General Hospital.

DISCLOSURE

The authors have nothing to disclose.

REFERENCES

1. Top 10 Chronic Conditions Affecting Older Adults. @NCOAging. Available at: https://www.ncoa.org/article/the-top-10-most-common-chronic-conditions-in-older-adults. Accessed January 14, 2023.

2. Demachkieh F, Lakissian Z, Kassab A, et al. Integrating palliative care for older adults: A needs assessment for Hamad Medical Corporation's geriatric services. Doha (Qatar): World Innovation Summit for Health; 2022.

3. Palliative care. Available at: https://www.who.int/news-room/fact-sheets/detail/palliative-care. Accessed January 15, 2023.

4. Lohman D, Callaway M, Pardy S, et al. Six key approaches in open society foundations' support for global palliative care development. J Pain Symptom Manage 2023;65(1):47–57.

5. Connor S. Launch of Qatar Palliative Care Needs Assessment for Older Persons. The Worldwide Hospice Palliative Care Alliance. Published October 5, 2022. Available at: http://www.thewhpca.org/2020-08-05-08-22-47/latest-news/item/launch-of-qatar-palliative-care-needs-assessment-for-older-persons. Accessed January 15, 2023.

6. The IHI Triple Aim | IHI - Institute for Healthcare Improvement. Available at: https://www.ihi.org/Engage/Initiatives/TripleAim/Pages/default.aspx. Accessed January 15, 2023.

7. Global Atlas of Palliative Care (2nd edition) - PAHO/WHO | Pan American Health Organization. Available at: https://www.paho.org/node/75063. Accessed January 15, 2023.

8. Global Ageing Network Presents at the United Nations. GlobalAgeing. Published August 1, 2018. Available at: https://globalageing.org/global-ageing-network-presents-at-the-united-nations/. Accessed January 15, 2023.

9. den Herder-van der Eerden M, van Wijngaarden J, Payne S, et al. Integrated palliative care is about professional networking rather than standardisation of care: a qualitative study with healthcare professionals in 19 integrated palliative care initiatives in five European countries. Palliat Med 2018;32(6):1091–102.

10. The Palliative Performance Scale (PPS). Palliative Care Network of Wisconsin. Available at: https://www.mypcnow.org/fast-fact/the-palliative-performance-scale-pps/. Accessed January 15, 2023.

11. Anderson F, Downing GM, Hill J, et al. Palliative performance scale (PPS): a new tool. J Palliat Care 1996;12(1):5–11.

12. Available at: https://www.mdcalc.com/calc/10426/g8-geriatric-screening-tool#use-cases. Accessed April 5, 2023.

13. What Is an Age-Friendly Health System? | IHI - Institute for Healthcare Improvemen. Available at: https://www.ihi.org:443/Engage/Initiatives/Age-Friendly-Health-Systems/Pages/default.aspx t. Accessed January 14, 2023.

14. Lowey SE. Withholding medical interventions and ageism during a pandemic: a model for resource allocation decision making. J Hospice Palliat Nurs 2021; 23(3):200.

15. Smith CB, Phillips T, Smith TJ. Using the new ASCO clinical practice guideline for palliative care concurrent with oncology care using the TEAM Approach. Am Soc Clin Oncol Educ Book 2017;37:714–23.

16. Sullivan DR, Chan B, Lapidus JA, et al. Association of early palliative care use with survival and place of death among patients with advanced lung cancer receiving care in the veterans health administration. JAMA Oncol 2019;5(12):1702–9.

17. Slavin SD, Warraich HJ. The right time for palliative care in heart failure: a review of critical moments for palliative care intervention. Rev Esp Cardiol Engl Ed 2020; 73(1):78–83.

18. Disler RT, Currow DC, Phillips JL, et al. Interventions to support a palliative care approach in patients with chronic obstructive pulmonary disease: an integrative review. Int J Nurs Stud 2012;49(11):1443–58.
19. Karam CY, Paganoni S, Joyce N, et al. Palliative care issues in amyotrophic lateral sclerosis: an evidenced-based review. Am J Hosp Palliat Care 2016;33(1):84–92.
20. Palliative Care and HIV/AIDS | Symptoms, Treatment | Get Palliative Care. Available at: https://getpalliativecare.org/whatis/disease-types/hivaids-palliative-care/. Accessed January 15, 2023.
21. Palliative care for people with dementia | British Medical Bulletin | Oxford Academic. Available at: https://academic.oup.com/bmb/article/96/1/159/299171. Accessed January 15, 2023.
22. Sternberg SA, Shinan-Altman S, Volicer L, et al. Palliative care in advanced dementia: comparison of strategies in three countries. Geriatr Basel Switz 2021; 6(2):44.
23. Hospice Around the World: Different Cultures, Different Views. Chapters Health System. Published October 28, 2021. Available at: https://www.chaptershealth. org/chapters-of-life-blog/families-caregivers/hospice-around-the-world-different-cultures-different-views/. Accessed January 15, 2023.
24. End-of-Life Care in an Aging World: A Global Perspective | American Academy of Actuaries. Available at: https://www.actuary.org/end-of-life-care. Accessed January 15, 2023.
25. Drenth C, Sithole Z, Pudule E, et al. Palliative care in South Africa. J Pain Symptom Manage 2018;55(2):S170–7.
26. Palliative Care Research in India - YouTube. Available at: https://www.youtube. com/watch?v=wNyAc90fjGY. Accessed January 14, 2023.
27. Howard. Palliative Care Toolkit (Nepali Edition) Launch. The Worldwide Hospice Palliative Care Alliance. Published August 23, 2022. Available at: http://www. thewhpca.org/2020-08-05-08-22-47/latest-news/item/palliative-care-toolkit-nepali-edition-launch. Accessed January 14, 2023.
28. Gomes B, de Brito M, de Lacerda AF, et al. Portugal needs to revolutionise end-of-life care. Lancet Lond Engl 2020;395(10223):495–6.
29. Special Report: Furthering Palliative Care Training in Latin America. Mass General Advances in Motion. Available at: https://advances.massgeneral.org/geriatrics/ journal.aspx?id=2358. Accessed January 15, 2023.
30. Putranto R, Mudjaddid E, Shatri H, et al. Development and challenges of palliative care in Indonesia: role of psychosomatic medicine. Biopsychosoc Med 2017;11:29.
31. Sithole Z, Dempers C. Palliative care in correctional centers-HPCA making progress in South Africa. J Pain Symptom Manage 2010;40(1):13–4.
32. Brant JM, Al-Zadjali M, Al-Sinawi F, et al. Palliative care nursing development in the Middle East and northeast Africa: lessons from Oman. J Cancer Educ 2021;36(Suppl 1):69–77.
33. The Lancet Commission on Palliative Care and Pain Relief—findings, recommendations, and future directions - The Lancet Global Health. Available at: https:// www.thelancet.com/journals/langlo/article/PIIS2214-109X(18)30082-2/fulltext. Accessed January 15, 2023.
34. Davila C, Cartagena L, Byrne-Martelli S, et al. Creating a dedicated palliative care team for ICU Spanish speaking patients in response to COVID-19. J Pain Symptom Manage 2022. https://doi.org/10.1016/j.jpainsymman.2022.12.013. S0885-3924(22)01045-4.

Printed and bound by CPI Group (UK) Ltd, Croydon, CR0 4YY

03/10/2024

01040466-0009